Pratap C Singhal MD'S

One Solution
To
Many Diseases

Presented

In

24 1/2 Inspirational Stories

Pratap C Singhal MD'S

One Solution
To
Many Diseases

Presented

In

24 1/2 Inspirational Stories

The disclaimer/warning
The chief message of these true stories in this book is to inspire and guide you for a better and healthier life, and it is not the objective to give you a personal advice, medical or non-medical, because there are so many individual variables. Therefore, you are advised to consult your physician before implementing any information in this book.

I have made every effort to make this book as accurate as possible. However, there still may be mistakes in the content or topography. Therefore, the author and the publisher shall assume no liability or responsibility, to any person or entity respect to any loss or damages caused or alleged to have been caused, directly or indirectly by the information contained in this book. Hence, the purchaser/reader must assume full responsibility for the use of the book or the information therein.

Invitation

By the Author

Hereby I invite you to take the challenge: Read the twenty-four and a half inspirational stories in this book with an open mind. I believe that most likely you will find the solution to your disease/condition. However, if you do not find then:

Do not run after the solution. You may get tired, exhausted or even faint. Rather sit down, relax (using the power of hypnosis and meditation/prayer), and have patience. Then let the solution will come to you spontaneously, painlessly, and effortlessly.

Pratap C Singhal MD

What others are saying. . .

In his book, *One Solution to Many Diseases,* Dr. Singhal displays the same evidence-based research and level of caring that he does in the hospital setting with his patients. At a time of an epidemic of obesity, hypertension, diabetes, and cholesterol issues, he offers a refreshingly different slant. Both clinician and layperson are guaranteed to find this helpful.

Frank J. Mazzarella, MD, CHCQM
Chief Medical Officer
Clara Maass Medical Center
Belleville, New Jersey

In the book, One Solution to Many Diseases, Dr. Singhal addresses the benefits of the disciplined healthy lifestyle and shows how it can help any patient. He also stresses the point that the benefits of weight loss are multiple that include: physical, mental, emotional, spiritual, and so on.

Senthamarai Gandhi, MD
Physician Advisor & Educator
Clara Maass Medical Center
Belleville, New Jersey

The author approaches the subject of one solution to many diseases from both practical and spiritual perspectives with an emphasis on long-term health and success.

Peter Gould, MD
Family Physician

This book by Dr. Singhal is indispensable for anybody. You must have a copy and use it as a manual and reference guide. Dr. Singhal has given us a method of healthier living, using mind and body in harmony.

Mathew J. DeLuca, MD
Neurologist

If you are interested in losing weight or addressing specific nutritional or medical concerns, I highly recommend this book by Dr. Singhal, *One Solution to Many Diseases*. You will definitely notice great results. The book is not just a diet but a total life changer.

Mercedes Macangay
Nursing Department Administrative Assistant

Dr. Singhal is a health and happiness coach who truly cares for his patients and the health profession. His research and information is done with love and care for people.

Roberta McKinney

As a patient of Dr. Singhal for thirty years, I feel that his caring, concern, and medical knowledge has transferred to his book. As everyone cannot be his patient because of location, I thoroughly recommend this book.

Karen Paglia

I have known Dr. Singhal for the past twelve years. I believe that he has the ability to change one's life when it comes to human health. Dr. Singhal is a renowned individual who takes other people's health seriously. His work speaks for itself. I believe that everyone should have Dr. Singhal as their family doctor, so that they can be better and enjoy life.

Ola Alade

One Solution to Many Diseases is packed with valuable information on weight loss and other health issues.

Diane Politano

Dr. Singhal's book, *One Solution to Many Diseases*, is very informative, and it will broaden your horizon. It will change your perspective on health and well-being.

Isabel Alves

If you want to make the process of health and well-being fun and enjoyable, you must read Dr. Singhal's book, *One Solution to Many Diseases*. You will love it.

Frank Ismaelito

Dr. Singhal is a physician who has demonstrated by medical case histories from his own practice how he has helped his patients to be healthier and happier when everything else had failed.

Fatimoh Alade
BSC Educational PSY

I have seen several books on weight loss; however, this book by Dr. Singhal is the simplest and easiest to follow.

Nina Ismaelito

I strongly believe that this is a handbook by Dr. Singhal, to a new and better you, is a must read.

Glenn Lahullier

Dr. Singhal teaches you a new way to be a healthier you.

Vivien L. Stewart

I have been a patient of Dr. Singhal for over twenty years. He always lifts up my spirit. He inspires self-confidence in me and counsels me on improving and maintaining my health.

James Feighery

Dr. Singhal has patience and a caring heart towards his patients. As a patient I was able to observe this through his treatment to me. "One Solution to Many Diseases" is very informative and useful for anybody at any time. It is an easy read because it is presented in short stories. It throws a lot of knowledge on various aspects of life concerning health and happy living.

Subba L. Maddipatla

Table of Contents

About the Author

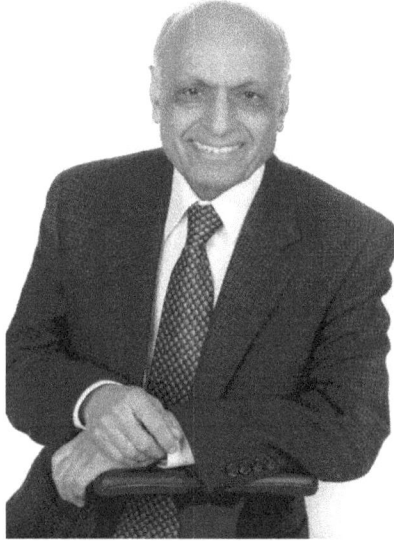

Pratap C Singhal MD practices conventional and complementary medicine. The field of complementary medicine includes homeopathy, hypnosis, and Maharishi Ayurveda and nutrition. He is also a stop-smoking specialist and a happiness coach. He has shared this multi-faceted expertise as a radio guest on several radio talk shows. He is the author of the book, *Health Happiness and You: Everything You Need to Know*, previously titled- *Live Healthier Live Happier* (with the help of 101-plus suggestions, formulas, poisons, mantras, and the lessons learned from short stories). He is working on a new book on cancer.

Dr. Singhal believes firmly that human life is very precious. Each human being has great potential and is responsible for his or her life's growth, development, high-rise and most importantly the physical and mental well-being. It is also the prime duty of every human being to continue to work toward this goal.

Acknowledgements

Six years ago, I wrote *Health Happiness and You: Everything You Need to Know*. The influx of testimonials has been a constant source of inspiration and encouragement for me to write this book. I appreciate your support and thank you very much.

I take this opportunity to thank those people who are responsible for the size, shape, and position I am in today.

Firstly, my mom and dad, the great souls: for their wisdom, love, care, for instilling in me the values of the human life, and for choosing me as their son. However, it may be possible that I chose them as my parents, or it could have been a mutual relationship.

To my wife Sushum: for encouraging me to study homeopathy and natural medicine, and for sharing the work and responsibility at home and work so that I can spend time for my book.

I am blessed with my three sons: Arun, Sunil, and Dhruv, and they are equally blessed with their spouses, namely, Monika, Sanchita, and Rebekka.

To my grandchildren, Kieran, Meera, Sonia, Sarin, Sarina and Kalyan, six of them at the time of writing this book: for being nothing but joy. The twinkle of their eyes and their energy, keeps me young and energized.

To my brothers and sisters and their spouses for being part of my life: one could not ask any better.

To all my friends and relatives: I have honored them in my first book and I honor them again here.

My special thanks to my two dear nephews, Vikram Singhal and Vivek Singhal: for their invaluable 24/7 support.

My very special thanks to my patients whose inspirational stories you will read in this book because they have shared them with an open heart and allowed me to publish them, without which this book could not have been possible.

I would like to acknowledge the Clara Maass Medical Center of Belleville New Jersey, a top-rated hospital in the United States of America with an excellent staff where I have treated most of my patients for last thirty years.

I would like to thank Mary Ellen Clyne, PhD, CEO of the hospital; Frank Mazzarella MD, CHCQMC; Senthamarai Gandhi MD; Peter Gould MD; Srinivasa Eswarapu MD; Patrick N. Ciccone MD; Keshav Shiva MD; Mehul N. Shah MD; and Matthew DeLuca MD for encouraging me to write this book.

I also thank Ms. Ritu Chopra, author, writer, speaker, and TV hostess for her encouragement.

Thank you to many of my patients who have become my friends over the years for their encouragement and interaction.

Finally, I must thank my secretary, Yerika Chavez, for her help with the manuscript, and Ms. Susan Giffin for her great job as editor of this book.

Most importantly, you the readers of this book: for giving me an opportunity to be part of your joy and well-being.

I would like to apologize to those whose names I might have missed inadvertently.

Thank you all very much.

Pratap C Singhal

Introduction

Dear Friends,

Congratulations for making the wise decision of investing in this book. I believe this book will turn out to be a life changer for you. You may wonder how there can be one solution to many diseases. It is easy once you analyze the phrase. One solution represents an awakened person. The un-awakened person has forgotten himself and his powers and therefore has become victim of many diseases. The awakened person with all his or her powers intact has been in existence ever since the creation of the human race and has been defeating all the diseases even when there was no medicine.

The awakened person is the solution to all the diseases. You will become more aware as you read the 24 ½ inspirational stories in this book. While reading these stories you will also enjoy the conversation that I'm having with the awakened person.

What brings the awakening to a person?
Many people are born with it, but in other cases it is a situational factor such as grief, sudden injury, and sudden realization that one has been traveling on the wrong path and in some cases it is the power of prayer, meditation and hypnosis and so on.

You will enjoy each story, but there are certain highlights in this book which I like to bring to your attention:

- *One Solution, One Script*: This is a very powerful script that I often use for my patients to bring some awakening. I believe it will also help you.

- *How a Cancer Patient Pulls Himself from Death's Door*: A lung cancer patient was laying in his death bed with only 35 days to live, when somehow his soul got the wake-up call. He made complete turnaround in his health. Within two months, he became cancer free. All by himself. **This is the power of the soul.**

- *Dealing with the Family Tragedy- Two Deaths in Matter of Minutes*: A heart breaking family tragedy where two loved ones died in a car accident. As a result, the surviving family members help each other to become stronger mentally and spiritually.

- *Stop Smoking in One Hour?* A smoker who repeatedly failed to quit smoking was heart-touched with the birth of his grandson. His soul aroused and then I was able to help him quit smoking in **one hour**.

- *I Wish to Die with Dignity and Peace.* It will demonstrate how the awakened person behaves at the time of his or her death.

- *The Best Healing Machine is Free*: The healing exercise that I have given in this chapter will aid your healing. You will use this exercise for rest of your life with benefits.

- *24 ½ Story*: This story is only half-finished. Attempt to finish with your own story. You will have fun, excitement and challenge with it.

There are many similar stories that relate to the power of hypnosis, they will all help you to become a stronger person, mentally and spiritually.

It gives me a great pleasure to share the stories with you as they have been not only inspiring but also an enriching experience for me as I was writing them. Finally, I hope these stories will also inspire and help you to move further in your life and you will also have the same fun and excitement with which I am presenting them here for you. I wish you all the best.

Sincerely,

Pratap C Singhal MD

One Solution, One Script

"You are there."

POEM

I'm giving you a special script.
If you know this script
You can be anything or have anything
I'm giving you a special script

People who know this script
Have made millions, and some even billions
Some have achieved the life of their dreams
This is the power of this goal setting script.
I'm giving you a special script

When I was a little boy
My mom gave me this script
Once my father saw me perplexed,
He reminded me of the same script
My teacher in school, and professor in college
All loved this goal setting script
They all used to say
You can be there, if you know your goal setting script.

I'm giving you a special script

They all told me again and again
They have been there
Many people have been there
You can also be there
If you know your goal-setting script

I'm giving you a special script

Here is the script
if you can just imagine
and if you could just dream
if you can be clear of your goal
and believe in yourself
then you can be anything and have anything
this is the goal setting script
'You are there' is the name of the script.

I'm giving you a special script

I have special advice
You must remember and practice the script
You must smile when you remember the script
Remember your script, in the morning, night
and also at all the time.
Then everywhere and in every way
the success will be yours.
This is the goal setting script

You are there, is the name of the script

I'm giving you a special script

This is the script, and the script is yours.
'You are there' is the name of this script
This is goal setting script.

I'm giving you a special script

Pratap C. Singhal MD

24 1/2

INSPIRATIONAL STORIES

Story 1

My Own Story:
A Transformation as a Medical Doctor

It was July, and the temperature must have been at least 95°F. My wife, my son, and I were at the railway station, waiting for the train. It was in the city of Hissar, India. All of a sudden, I was seized by the acute onset of excruciating pain in my belly, and I was in agony. Almost ten to fifteen people gathered around me in sympathy, and they were saying that I had a real colic.

The train that we had been waiting for came and left, and, thank goodness, we did not take the train. The reason why we were at the train station was that my wife and I had planned a one-week vacation which was long overdue. My wife, my son, and I had been all excited and thrilled, but this excruciating pain in my belly changed everything. Now the excitement and joy changed to uncertainty and sadness.

The stationmaster came to us after hearing all the commotion. To him, it was nothing new, and it did not take him much to understand the situation. He immediately called the ambulance and stayed there till they picked me up to take to the hospital.

The ambulance on its route to the hospital had the siren on so that they could get the right-of-way. I was in the hospital in matter of minutes.

This was the same hospital where I was employed. In my own

hospital, my own staff gave me VIP treatment, including a private room. I had just left the hospital only a couple of hours earlier after making rounds and finishing the clinic. I had told them I was going away for one week and when I returned, I would be fully energized and rejuvenated. But I came back only after a couple of hours later as a patient. Some nurses said jokingly, "We did not expect you this soon."

The doctor in charge of the hospital came to see me immediately. I was told I had a kidney stone and urinary tract infection. It was his clinical diagnosis, and no x-rays were taken or ultrasound done. This is the way it was done in those days [1968], at least in that hospital setting. Everything was clinical, and if the patient did not get better, he or she was transferred to a district hospital.

After the doctor examined me, he prescribed pain medication and antibiotics. This was the same hospital where I used to give orders to the nurses on daily basis, but today things are different. Today I was a patient. Today the nurses were telling me what to do, what not to do, what I could eat, and so on. They also advised me that I could get pain medication every four hours, if needed.

I was in the hospital for approximately six days. The regiment of antibiotic and pain medication was not helping me, and I was getting worse by the day. I had lost my appetite and was losing weight. The thought or the smell of food would make me throw up. I was feeling cold in the hot month of July and was sweating profusely, and it was offensive. I do not know about others, but my wife and my son did not care about the offensiveness of the sweat. My wife and I both were getting nervous, concerned, desperate, and even confused as what to do next.

A new hope: It was my sixth day in the hospital, Thursday evening around 6:00 p.m. when one of my friends came to visit me. He was a homeopathic doctor. He advised and assured me that I should seek homeopathic treatment that would cure my condition, but he also told me that this was not within his scope of work. This information was a blessing. We felt as if a new hope had arrived from heaven.

The next morning, my wife planned a trip to meet and consult a great homeopathic doctor. It was an eighty-mile trip. It would take twelve hours for the round-trip by the bus. My wife decided that I should not be left alone, so she left my three-year-old boy to stay with me. During my six days of stay at the hospital, most of the nurses had become friendly with my son and my wife. My wife also told the nurses that she was leaving our son there so that he can call them in case my husband needed some help. She also told my son, "If Daddy has pain, go get the nurse and tell her my daddy needs something for pain."

Before leaving for her trip, she fed my son breakfast, and arranged snacks and toys for him. She also arranged for lunch to be delivered at noontime from a nearby hotel.

For the long twelve hours from 7:00 a.m. to 7:00 p.m. when my wife was gone, my son and I were the best partners. He would often ask me, "Daddy, if you have pain, just let me know. I will call the nurse." I was thinking the other way around, how my little son was stuck at the hospital. I did my best to keep him busy and entertained for those hours. I would ask him often if he was hungry. "There are snacks for you, and if you are tired, you can lie down. If you want to play there are toys for you, or if you want to draw, there is a drawing book for you." And so on.

His lunch arrived at noon as scheduled, and I told him to take his lunch. You know that the thought and the smell of food used to make me throw up, but that day it did not. Rather, I enjoyed watching him eat his lunch.

My wife came back at 7:00 p.m., exactly twelve hours after she had left. She had a smile on her face and was hopeful. She said the homeopathic doctor told her to bring her husband as soon as possible; he shall wait for us. I had been a very positive person to start with, so I also became hopeful.

On Saturday morning, we left the hospital around 8:00 a.m. by a taxi that my wife had arranged. It was a six-hour long journey. The roads were not that great those days, and there were many bumps, some small and some big. My wife had made me lie down in the back seat of the taxi. She put my head in her lap, and my son sat at the end by my feet. I felt every bump, small or big, because my body had become very sensitive to pain. Every bump did its best to test me, and with every bump I would moan with pain.

My wife kept comforting and consoling me throughout the journey, saying that we should be there soon, and it is not that far.

With every moan, my son would look at me first and then at his mother with the feeling of helplessness, and then he would turn his head away. Finally, we completed the long, six-hour journey.

As soon as our taxi arrived, the homeopathic doctor was informed. He came out of the class that he had been teaching. He asked my wife to get out of the taxi, and he took her seat. He put my head in his lap and asked me two questions. These questions imprinted on me, and I still remember them as if yesterday.

His first question was, "Where is the pain?"

I told him that the pain is in my right kidneys, and I pointed to them with my fingers.

Next, he asked me, "Can I squeeze your belly?"

I yelled loudly, "No, my belly is very sensitive."

Then he left me to fetch some medicine. He came back in few minutes and poured ten to fifteen very tiny pellets into my mouth and asked me do not swallow them; just let them dissolve in my mouth slowly.

Next, two magical thing happened in matter of minutes.

Firstly, within two minutes, my pain was gone for good. I could not believe how the pain could have disappeared that fast. I squeezed my belly everywhere over and over again to test if this is true and indeed it was true. I felt as if God has touched me or some miracle has happened. I still could not believe it, and I kept looking at my wife, my son, and the doctor back and forth. Of course, the doctor was very pleased with my progress. My wife and my son were equally amazed; they could not get over it. They also kept looking at the doctor and me over and over again.

The second magical thing was that I felt hungry within fifteen minutes. Up until that time, the thought or smell of food had made me want to throw up, but now I wanted to eat something.

[You may be aware of the fact that returning to an appetite is one of the important signs of healing.]

Next, the doctor's wife made some pudding for me because there was no place to cook. I ate that pudding in matter of minutes, and I could not express how strong I felt after eating it. I felt I had regained my energy and was almost normal.

We stayed overnight at the college campus. The doctor told me that he wanted to observe me, so I needed to stay there for that night. This was the first night that I could not sleep because till then, I was able to sleep in the hospital under the effect of pain medications, but this night I could not sleep because I was excited and could not believe or understand how a few pellets of homeopathic remedy could cure my condition in matter of a few minutes. Also I kept thinking as to why the conventional medicine that I practiced had failed to cure my condition. I felt ignorant as to how little I knew about the medical science of healing.

However, this was a different situation with my wife. This was the first night that she had had a good night's sleep because now she had no more worries about me. She had been exhausted from watching me over for one week in the hospital.

For your information, most people know that in conventional

medicine, treatment is based on the diagnosis. As I had been diagnosed with having kidney stones and infection, I was treated with antibiotics for infection and morphine for pain. However, in homeopathy, it is a multiple prong or a global approach. In homeopathy, the fact that I had pain and infection was taken into the consideration, but the second fact, which was more important than the first one, was how I was reacting to my illness. The fact I stated, "Do not touch me because I'm very sensitive" helped the homeopathic doctor to prescribe me the homeopathic remedy.

However, if I had stated that I was very sore, and please rub it or apply heat to it, I would have received a different remedy.

Let me give you another example. If a patient would yell and scream at the time of presenting his or her condition, the remedy would be totally different, even with the same medical diagnosis or condition.

My life has been transformed for good.

The incident of renal colic—not responding to the conventional treatment and responding so dramatically to the homeopathic treatment—was a unique combination that brought the change in my thinking process. I became aware of the fact that something was missing in the healing medicine that I had been practicing.

I was impressed with the science of homeopathy that had saved my life. Up till that time, like most other doctors, I had no respect for homeopathy or any other complementary branches of healing;

however, now it was a total turnaround in my opinion. As you all know, things are changing today. Doctors and people are more open to the complementary branches of healing, including homeopathy. I have noticed that many surgeons use a homeopathic remedy—Arnica Montana—routinely for the postoperative pain, and hospitals have accepted that.

A conflict was going on in my mind. The next day, we left the homeopathic doctor with his consent. I had millions of thoughts about what I should do or should not do. Should I go back to my previous job where I treated my patients with conventional medicine or should I explore and study the science of homeopathy that had saved my life? It was a quite a struggle in my mind. Finally, the second thought won, and I made up my mind to study homeopathy. I went back to the hospital and took a leave of absence for the purpose of studying homeopathy.

My belief was further affirmed by one another incident. During my wife's pregnancy, she started to bleed from her rectum. She was seven-and-a-half months pregnant at the time. I took her to her obstetrician who recommended that the best thing for her was bed rest until the time of delivery. Nothing surgical should be done because it may not be good for the pregnancy. However, because of my new insight into homeopathy, I consulted a physician who practiced complementary medicine. He prescribed a remedy that stopped her bleeding and she did not have to stay in bed. This second incident further deepened my belief in homeopathy.

The more I studied the science of homeopathy, the more

respect I developed for this healing science. Now my mind was open to anything. I was ready to explore other branches of healing. Thereafter, I also studied hypnosis (the science of healing using the conscious and subconscious mind), Ayurveda (the science of life), self-healing (making the self-effort by using one's own knowledge), and nutrition (the food for the body and the mind). Ever since then, I have used these modalities in my practice and have been quite impressed with their effectiveness. Today, as the result of this transformation, I have much more to offer to my patients than just conventional medicine, which was my only tool before my sickness.

My sickness had made me realize how determined and courageous my wife was. I thank her for her persistence.

My father's usual statement had come true. He used to say, "Keep your eyes and ears open. No matter how much you know; there's a lot more to know."

Let me conclude my story with this statement. The art of healing sciences has several branches, including, conventional medicine, homeopathy, hypnosis, Ayurveda, nutrition, and others. All healing sciences have something unique to offer, and every healing science has some limitations and gaps. Fortunately, gap left by one healing science can be filled by another. I believe that people should keep their mind and eyes open and should take advantages of these complementary healing sciences, if and when they are needed.

My sickness experience broadened my mental horizon, and, most importantly, it made me a better doctor and a better human being that has affected the lives of many of my patients as well as of mine.

Some people may wonder why I started this book with my own story. There are a couple of reasons.

Firstly, I wanted to set a precedent for those patients who have been kind enough to allow me to share their stories in this book. I want them to know that sharing is a good thing if it helps someone else. Secondly, my story is an example of a transformation of my life as a medical doctor. I believe the disease was sent by God to put me in the right path.

In 2010, I wrote the book, *Health Happiness and You – Everything You Need to Know*. This book was also published under the different title, *Live Healthier, Live Happier* – With the help of 101+ suggestions, formulas, poems, mantras, and lessons learned from short stories. This book is the product of that transformation of my life as a human being and as a physician. In this book, I have devoted at least one hundred pages so that people can learn to heal themselves.

Story 2

Hypnotize Me, Please!

One Friday evening, before the end of the day, my secretary told me that I had one last patient. As I entered the examining room, I saw a woman in her mid-thirties.

"Hello, I'm Dr. Singhal."

"I'm Holly," she said.

"How can I help you?"

"Please hypnotize me!" she said.

When I heard those words, *hypnotize me*, I got energized. On that Friday, I had a long day, and I was getting tired, but the words *hypnotize me* restored my energy.

From my experience, when people come to me for any complementary science of healing such as hypnosis, homeopathy, Ayurveda, and so on, I get energized. There are a couple of reasons to that. The first and foremost reason is that these people expect more from me, and, fortunately, I can offer them more versus than when someone comes for conventional treatment. That also makes the visit more challenging and interesting. Secondly, in most cases if not all, these people have tried other modalities of treatment unsuccessfully and are looking for an alternative or complementary modality of healing.

"Why do you want to be hypnotized?" I asked her.

She replied, "Because I want to lose weight."

It is an important question to ask why people want to be hypnotized because hypnosis can be used for multiple purposes or conditions beside weight loss. For example, it can be used to stop smoking, manage anger or stress, the fear of the dentist, deter panic attacks, and so on. Therefore, it is important for the practitioner to clarify the goal of the patient in the very beginning.

Next I asked her, "How much weight do you want to lose?"

She replied, "Thirty pounds, and I must lose them in four months, so I don't have much time." She also told me she does not like the idea of fasting because she would die without food. (Unfortunately, some people think that you can die of fasting; however, that is not true.)

At this juncture, I asked how she chose the services of my office. She said, "You have treated one of my sister's friends who lost thirty pounds in three months, and she is quite happy with that. I also learned from your book that you are a hypnotherapist as well as a physician, so I can trust you. Otherwise I'm afraid of hypnosis."

Next, I explained to her that I could hypnotize her to lose weight, but she had to come for four to five sessions, depending how much progress she makes. She agreed. Thereafter, I set her first appointment for three days later, based upon the schedule and availability.

First session: Holly showed up for her first scheduled appointment for hypnosis.

In order to understand the cause of obesity, I asked her many questions, and from her response, I learned that she has problem with overeating, and she also snacks often. She does not like fruits and vegetables, and she loves meat. She also takes dessert before bedtime and does not exercise.

On examination: Holly is forty-seven years old. She stands 5'3" and weighs 235 pounds. Her blood pressure is 140/90. She does not smoke or drink.

She has no medical problems and does not take any medication. She had had no surgeries in the past. She is a college graduate, a teacher, and the mother of three children. She's very pleasant, intelligent, and successful woman. She is well-dressed; however, she's kind of embarrassed because of her weight.

I gave her a blood test to make sure that she has no diabetes or cholesterol issues, and to make sure that she does not have any problem with kidneys, liver, or thyroid glands.

At this juncture, I asked her tell me more about herself and what made her decide to lose weight?

Holly had a very interesting story to tell, so I want you to read her story in her own language. She continues:

> I am a successful woman, and I have a great husband and three children. I come from a big family. I am a role model in the opinion of all my family members because of my success not only at work but also at home. Therefore my friends and family seek my advice about everything.
>
> Two weeks ago, my sister told me that she was planning a family reunion in the month of July, just four months from now. My sister painted a rosy picture of the whole program. She told me that reunion would

take place on a beach where everybody would have bikinis and swimsuits. Initially, I became very happy, but all of a sudden my heart started to sink, even when I was on the phone with her. I became aware of my weight and thought how I would look in a bikini or swimsuit. I felt blah. My belly is hanging, and my legs are fat, and none of my old swimsuits fit me.

"I have tried to lose weight in the past, but always it was like a yo-yo. But now I have made up my mind. I am willing to do anything. I have only four months to go."

Next, I gave her information about healthy eating. I also stressed upon her the many important elements, namely that she stop snacking and cut down the portion sizes of her meals. I also advised her to cut down all rich and fatty foods, especially meat, desserts, and sodas, and also to increase her intake of water-rich food (fruits, vegetables and soups). I stressed the importance of exercise and advised that she must start some kind of exercise program. I advised her to monitor her weight regularly and keep a log of it, and that she should bring it with her on each visit for my review so that I can understand her better. Finally, I advised her to keep a food diary of each and every thing that she ate, so I could understand her eating habits and behavior.

In order to prepare her for hypnosis, I had to remove some common myths about hypnosis. She was assured that hypnosis is a safe and effective modality. I told her that people do not get stuck in hypnosis as some people rumor. I also assured her that nobody including myself would be able to control her during the state of hypnosis. Finally, I asked, "Are you ready for hypnosis?"

She replied, "Yes."

Next, I hypnotized her and taught her self-hypnosis. I told her to practice this help self-hypnosis for a week and then come back for her next weight loss session.

Second session: Holly returned for her second scheduled session. I asked her how she is doing with self-hypnosis. She replied she was doing well and enjoying it. She also told me that hypnosis makes her relax.

After hypnotizing her, I told her the following:

> "Holly, close your eyes. Imagine as vividly as possibly you can and believe with your heart and soul that you have lost thirty-five pounds. Your body is perfect, just as you want it to be. This is your new body, the body of your dreams. If you like, you can touch and feel it. You can feel your long neck, tucked-in belly, firm and smooth legs—all in your wildest imagination and make it as vivid as you can. Also imagine that now you are at the beach at the family reunion, and everybody is watching you and admiring what you have achieved in the last four months.
>
> "You are happy, excited and thrilled. You cannot believe how you have lost so much weight and how good you look and feel. You cannot stop looking at yourself in the mirror, and you take pride in yourself. You are agile and active. You want to tell the whole world what you have achieved in the last few months. Your husband loves you more now than ever before, and your colleagues also admire you.
>
> "If you would like to hear somebody describing how good you look, imagine an artist describing your body to you in details and pay attention to the every word the artist says.

"You can stay at this stage of vivid imagination till you are 100 percent convinced that everything is real and you have lost all that weight. Thereafter, you can open your eyes."

After my last statement, she stayed in the state of hypnosis for additional seven minutes and then opened her eyes with the feeling of amazement and kept looking at me and said it feels good.

I took her off hypnosis. Next I told her, "Since this script is very important, and you are going to use on daily basis, let us name this goal-setting script 'You are there.'"

I gave her the copy of the script to follow at home. I explained to her that there are few important things that she needed to remember about this script.

Firstly, this script needs to be practiced very frequently, as often as twenty, thirty, even forty times a day. Initially, it may take two to three minutes with each exercise, but with the practice it should not take more than five to ten seconds. Otherwise, it is not possible to do so often.

She was also advised that the second most important element is the smile. She must smile before and after each goal-setting exercise because when she smiles, she gets in touch with her inner self and that creates an awakening or awareness within her that has a deeper and longer-lasting effect.

I explained to her that the best way to start is to do the exercise every half hour from the time she gets up till the time she goes to bed. She should also do this exercise before and after each meal, before and after each shower, and also before and after dressing and undressing, and so on.

Next, I gave an appointment for the third session after one week.

Third session: In this session, I asked her how she had been doing with this script and hypnosis. She said she is very pleased and has lost two pounds. But most importantly, she said that now she felt that she had a grip on her dietary habits and was confident she could do it.

I continued to follow Holly for four months. She lost thirty-seven pounds. She was excited and thrilled with the progress she had made. In fact, she lost more than she had wanted to lose. I congratulated her, and she cried out of joy and thanked me.

Before concluding this chapter, let me say a few words about the power of this goal-setting script, "You are there."

This script is extremely powerful and has changed the lives of many, including myself. I can assure you that if you will use this script, you will be amazed and happy with the results. It is extremely important to know that you must be clear in your goal before you use this goal-setting script, and of course you have to modify it a little, based on your needs and expectations.

Next let me show you how this script helped me to become a doctor. After graduating from college, I entered medical school in 1959. It was a five-year program.

It was extremely hard to get into medical school. Furthermore, I knew it was a very tough and challenging program to go through, and I was nervous and apprehensive like everyone else because many people dropped out of the program. I was constantly asking myself if I could survive the program. I did not have much support because I did not have many friends; I used to be very shy. My parents and family were my only support, but I did not see them often because I was in a boarding school. I saw them only when I went home; however, they did their best to give me the support and encouragement on an ongoing basis.

The first day I went to medical school, the nurses, paramedical staff, even professors started to call me doctor. This was the way it was. The day the students entered medical school, they are labeled doctors, and there is a purpose behind it. The students are made to think, act, and behave like a doctor. They are advised that they must learn to lift themselves emotionally and intellectually. As you know, the word doctor is a very powerful, at least to a first-year medical student who does not know even a word of medicine or disease. But I was labeled as a doctor on the very first day of medical school, and as I kept hearing the word doctor day after day, it helped me to lift up myself enough to get through five long, tough years of medical school until I graduated and got my license.

Such is the power of the script.

I think you can fall in love with this script if you use it.

Let me suggest here that it is a good time for you to refresh your memory with the script 'You are there' (poem) that appears at the beginning of this book.

Story 3

The Dedication of a Mother

Sandy was in my office for her fifth regular yearly physical. This was the first year that she was happy and excited for the physical and had a smile on her face. (In the past years, she used to be sad and complain about her weight at every physical.) I asked her, "Sandy, tell me what makes you so happy."

She told me, "You will find it out soon and you will be proud of me because I have lost more than thirty-five pounds since last year. I bet my cholesterol level and hemoglobin A-1 C level will be good. Just give me good checkup."

Sandy is 35 years old and 5' tall. Today she weighs 185 pounds; however, for the last five years her weight had been stagnant at 215 pounds. Today her blood pressure was 120/80, but in the past, it had been always borderline high, ranging from 130 to 140/85 to 90. She does not smoke or drink. She is a housewife and very loving and caring person. She has two children, Tony and Willie, and both of her children are overweight.

I gave her a full physical and then gave her a blood test. I was surprised that this is the first time that her cholesterol was normal and so was her hemoglobin A-1 C. I told her, "Sandy, this is the best physical you have had in last five years."

She started to look into my eyes with pride and accomplishment. She asked me, "Do you really want to know the whole story?"

"Yes, of course."

Sandy told her story:

"One day, I received a call from one of my children at school that I should come to the school to meet my son Tony's teacher. I went to the school very nervous and anxious, wondering what had happened to my son.

"Tony's teacher was very sympathetic in her words and tone. She told me that Tony's weight was affecting him negatively. 'He cannot keep up with his peers and cannot play without getting short of breath. Many times he feels so embarrassed that he refuses to play. As you know, his grades are falling, and this is not good for his emotional and intellectual growth. If I were you, I would take him to his doctor.'

"I told the teacher, 'Thank you very much. I appreciate your bringing this information to my awareness. You have opened my eyes, and I can put two and two together.

"Today I can understand why Tony has been less interested in his school and studies. Before, he used to love school. I had asked Tony few times why he no longer enjoys school. He would shrug his shoulders and walk away, or he simply say, "Johnny or Suzy don't like me." I could not put two and two together. I thought it was children's stuff, but today everything is making sense.

"It was Friday afternoon the start of a long weekend. I called his pediatrician immediately as soon as I left the school. Fortunately, the pediatrician had evening hours and could see my son the same day. I took a sigh of relief that I did not have to spend a long weekend in anxiety of waiting.

"The pediatrician examined Tony. He told me that Tony weighed 165 pounds, at least 60 pounds overweight. He also told me that he had a touch of high blood pressure. His blood sugar and cholesterol are also slightly high. The pediatrician told me that

Tony gets short of breath easily. He also cautioned that it is not a good situation for Tony and not good for his mental and emotional growth. The pediatrician told me that Tony must lose weight and that if he does not, most likely he will be an overweight adult. I became extremely apprehensive when I heard the words hypertension and diabetes because my husband also suffers from these conditions.

"I asked him where to start because I was so nervous and overwhelmed. He explained to me that the most important thing was for Tony to reduce his meal portion sizes and start exercising, and this would be a good start. He also gave me literature on obesity and a list of certain websites for more information. He also recommended that I see the nutritionist.

"I started to think how I could motivate my children. I kept thinking on this issue over and over, and finally, **I came to the conclusion that the best way to motivate my children would be to set an example. I needed to become a role model for them. In that way it would be easier for them**.

"Next I turned everything around in my home. Now that my mind was set, I must bring change at home and became health-conscious. I made sure that I served smaller portions of food at mealtime and ate less. I also made sure there were plenty of fruits and vegetables at home. I made sure the children exercised regularly, and I joined them as they were exercising. When the children would ask for a snack, I will offer them a fruit rather than dessert. If children would ask for soda, I will offer them water, juice or smoothie.

"And if children wanted to go out, I made sure they made healthy choices or encouraged them to eat home where I made sure that I served healthy meals. I stopped buying TV dinners and became 100 percent committed and determined.

"I also realized that change is not easy, so I became closer to them than ever before. I started to spend more time with them and started to show more love. Many times, I read stories to them at bedtime that I never had done before. I realized that because of my bonding, they were more open to accept changes than ever before.

"Three months later, my son Tony had lost thirty pounds. I took him back to his doctor for a checkup. The doctor told me that Tony had no more touch of diabetes. His cholesterol is normal and so was his blood pressure. I became ecstatic.

"Believe it or not, it also changed my life. I have also lost thirty-five pounds along with my other two children because I had done the same I was teaching my children. I always believed that the best way to motivate someone is to set an example and to become a role model. I'm aware that it requires dedication and sacrifices, but for me it is a small price to pay for the sake of my children. I would do anything for my children.

"This incident had brought a transformation in my family and also has brought my family closer to each other than before. In reality, it has been a rewarding experience in many ways—for me and for my family.

"I am very glad about what I did for them. I have come to the realization that the cause of my obesity was the unhealthy lifestyle with which my parents have brought me up, although they did mean well. Since they had seen rough days in their lives, they wanted to make sure that we always had plenty of food at home. **Excess food, instead of being a boon, became a curse. Today I am proud that I have given my children the gift of a healthy lifestyle. I hope they will continue the same and set an example for their children."**

Story 4

The Lady Who Traveled 70 Miles Daily to My Clinic

On a sunny afternoon, I was in my clinic, seeing my patients regularly but as I entered one of the examining rooms, I saw a former patient of mine that I had not seen for more than ten years. Her name is Tammy. She used to live in the town where I have an active practice at the present time. However, because of the job situation, she had moved seventy miles south.

In amazement, I asked her, "How are you, Tammy?"

She replied, "I feel awful. I know I have not seen you for a very long time." All of a sudden, she had tears in her eyes. Tammy is a very emotional person, so I was not surprised about her reaction.

Going further, I asked her, "How can I help you?"

Tammy began explaining the ongoing issues of her weight. She said, again with tears in her eyes,

> "I am fat and ugly. How I can get rid of this weight? I have been dating for five years. Last week, my boyfriend asked me to marry him. I became excited and thrilled, but when I went home, I cried for hours. I began to ask myself, 'How ugly do I look at this weight, and how will any wedding dress fit me?'
>
> "Although I know I have been overweight, but I had never paid any attention to it, but this incident has created an awareness that I need to do something for my weight."

I asked Tammy, "What made you decide to come to see me after so many years?"

"I had read the chapter about fasting in your book, *Health Happiness and You – Everything You Need to Know.* In this chapter, you mentioned that fasting is the best way to lose weight quickly and naturally. After reading the chapter, I did lot of research on Internet, and I think fasting is for me, so I'm here.

In order to confirm, I asked her again, "So, you want to go on fasting?"

She replied, "Yes, that's what I want, and I would like you to supervise me during the process of fasting."

Next I asked her, "How much weight do you want to lose?"

"At least thirty pounds."

"How much time do you have?"

She said, "Not much. I need to lose weight as quickly as possible because I think no dress will look good on me in this weight."

I told Tammy, "Yes, I agree with you. In this case, fasting is your best option."

She also told me that she had pretty good understanding about fasting because she had done her homework.

Next, I asked her, "Do you have any previous experience in fasting?"

She replied, "No."

I cautioned her that in that case, she needed to come to see me every day or at the most every other day. "Is it possible for you since you live seventy miles away?"

"Yes, I will travel seventy miles per day, if I have to. Now that my mind is set, I am ready to do anything because I need help badly."

At this juncture, I agreed to supervise her during the period of fasting, and she smiled in acceptance.

Next I took her history and examined her.

Tammy is forty-five years old, 5'4", 253 pounds. (Her ideal weight would have been 130–140 pounds. Her blood pressure is 120/85 and pulse is 85 minute. She is single and has no children. She has no medical condition and no surgeries in the past. She does not smoke or drink and has no allergies. She has a degree in psychology and works in the hospital as a caseworker. She likes to socialize a lot, and therefore she has a lot of friends.

After examination, I gave her a blood test. She has no evidence of diabetes or cholesterol. Her vitamin D was normal, and so were the thyroid function tests. Her kidneys and liver functions were also normal. I discussed all the blood report findings with her and assured her that her blood test was normal.

In preparation for fasting, I cautioned her that because fasting is a commitment, she might feel little weak for a day or so, only in the beginning of the fasting process. However, I also assured her that thereafter she should be fine. She said that she was ready for anything.

I also advised her not to eat or drink anything except water during the entire duration of fasting. She told me she was aware of that. I told her that she could continue to do her work; there was no need to take time off. However, I advised her not to exercise, and she agreed to that. I saw her on Thursday and advised her to start fasting on Sunday. I gave her an appointment to see me on Monday, i.e., twenty-four hours after she started her fast.

Tammy came back Monday for her second visit. She has been fasting for twenty-four hours. She was in good physical and mental condition except complaints of little weakness. (It is quite typical of fasting experience that people feel weak in first twenty-four to forty-eight hours.)

On examination, I found that now she weighs 251 pounds. She had lost two pounds. Her blood pressure is slightly low at 115/80. Her pulse is 65, which is also slightly low. She's slightly dehydrated. Her blood test shows that she has no abnormality of the kidney or liver, and her blood sugar is normal.

I told her do not worry about weakness, just keep well hydrated and she would be fine. I have learned from experience that during the periods of fasting, dehydration is one of the important causes of weakness. I also advised her that now that her body is going into anaerobic metabolism, it has healing effect on her mind and body, and of course she will continue to lose weight. Next, I assured her that if she has any questions, she should free to call me 24/7; otherwise I will see her back in two days, i.e., Wednesday.

I saw Tammy on Wednesday for the third time. Again she was looking good physically and emotionally. She has lost three and a half more pounds from the previous visit. She told me she is urinating a lot, and her weakness is gone. Her blood pressure has dropped to 110/75, and her pulse has also dropped to 60. She has been working as usual. Her blood test was again within normal limits. I encouraged her to keep on fasting. I also advised her that any time she does not feel comfortable, she can break the fast with a glass of juice. I reminded her how important it is to keep hydrated. I gave her permission to call me any time if she has any question or concern. We set her next follow-up appointment in another two days.

This process continued for twenty-one days. On her last visit, she had lost total of twenty-seven pounds. She told me, "I'm ready for a piece of toast." I congratulated her and she thanked me.

She also had tears in her eyes, but these tears were quite different. They were of joy and accomplishment, not like the initial tears of helplessness.

She also commented before leaving, "It was not as difficult as I thought. Now food does not control me. I am in charge, and this is the way it is going to be." She then asked me one question before leaving, "Can I do it again?"

I told her, "Of course! This is the most beautiful part of the program. If you do it once, you can do it again and again. Each and every subsequent act of fasting becomes easier and easier." I also told her that most likely she would not need my help in this reference, however if she does, I would be available for her.

I was amazed with her accomplishment. I cannot say for sure whether she had been such a strong person initially or if fasting made her so, or it may be a combination of both.

In reference to fasting, let me stress one point: Fasting is one of the best, cheapest, and most natural modality to lose weight quickly without side effects. However, one needs to be supervised during the period of fasting. Fasting is not used just for weight loss but also to strengthen physical, mental, emotional, and spiritual elements of the being.

One also needs to know that during the period of water fasting, the person is not allowed to take any food or beverage except water. Fasting is quite a common practice among many religions. There are various modified ways of fasting; for example, some people go on milk fast, while others do fruit fast, and so on.

There is one misconception about fasting. Some patients of mine have asked me, "Can you die of fasting?"

I say emphatically, "No, you cannot die of fasting." Fasting is not starvation, nor is starvation fasting. During fasting, you have the choice to break the fast whenever you wish or need to do so. Fasting is very safe, cheap, and effective modality. One also needs to know that one may often complain of weakness in the first or second day, but experience has shown that weakness disappears very shortly thereafter; one of the important causes of weakness is dehydration.

A word of caution: Fasting, if done too often and for a prolonged period of time, can cause malnutrition.

People who are old or underweight also have to be extremely careful. They must not fast without strict supervision.

Story 5

Two Medical Residents – Two Stars

One Sunday evening, it was raining so heavily you could hear the soothing sound of falling rain from the partially open window. Four resident doctors were sitting in the medical residents' lounge, trying to make up their schedule for the following week.

A lot of things happen at the medical residents' lounge. Here, most residents come and go every now and then for a few minutes or so to relax, if they can find the time. Very often, you hear a resident complaining of the heavy schedule which is hard on the body and the mind. (You might not know that during my time as a resident, we used to work sixteen to eighteen hours a day and also weekends, which was quite normal.)

Some resident tell his true heroic story that he had not urinated for twelve hours because he could not leave the clinic for a minute, and his bladder was ready to burst. The other resident might say he did not have the chance to take a bite of food for twelve hours, and he was ready to faint. The most common complaint is not sleeping for twenty-four hours or even thirty-six hours. These situations were not uncommon, but things are changing now.

In the lounge, residents often discussed difficult and challenging cases and tried to make use of the experiences of one another. At times, the discussion became heated, and the residents started to yell at each other for missing a diagnosis or not doing a test in a timely manner. In the medical field, the seniors often point out the mistakes of the residents without any hesitation. Many residents feel that it is degrading; however, this is an accepted practice in the medical community. They say that maybe it is better to learn this way than the hard way. You may also want to know that some of the attending physicians or teachers can be quite hard on their residents, and that adds to the stress.

Anyhow, as we were discussing the schedule, the TV was on. (For your information, in the doctors' lounge, the TV never goes off.) There was a program on the TV about obesity. The purpose of the program was to create **public awareness** about obesity, how the obesity can contribute or be the cause of multiple problems or conditions, such as diabetes, high blood pressure, heart disease, arthritis, cholesterol issues, and so on. Obesity even puts one at the increased risk of certain cancers.

All of a sudden, one resident (Dr. B) said, "I think I am getting fat. At present, I weigh 227 pounds, and I need to lose at least 40 pounds. Up till now, I had never given a thought that obesity could cause diabetes. Now I remember that my father was told to lose weight as he was diabetic."

The second resident (Dr. K) said, "Yes, I agree. I also need to lose at least thirty pounds as I am also getting out of shape."

Before you knew it, both were looking at each other as if to get some kind of agreement from each other. All of a sudden, both simultaneously said, "Let us lose weight," and they shook hands in confirmation. Both residents had set their minds to losing weight and becoming healthy.

Next Dr. B said, "Let us make it fun and challenging," and Dr. K agreed.

Dr. B said, "Today is November 3. There are twenty-seven days left in this month. Let us say whosoever loses more weight by the end of the month will be in the winner. And the loser has to treat the winner to dinner." Thereafter, both shook hands and the bet was on. This is a pretty good bet, considering the salary a resident used to earn.

The third resident, who was also fat, shrugged his shoulders and said, "I don't want to be part of it," and left. However, I stayed and enjoyed the process. I was not fat, so I did not have to lose any weight.

As you might already know, medical residents are a very important part of any hospital. There are several reasons for that. Let me give you two of the most common ones. Firstly, residents are in the hospital 24/7. They know each and every nurse, technician, administrator, and attending physician. And, of course, most of the patients know them. Secondly, residents are there to help not only the patients but also the nurses and staff. For example, if there is an emergency and the attending physician could not come, the resident takes over the case. It is a good system that works in favor of the patients and everyone else; such is the importance of the residents.

Now, let us return to the story of the two residents who made a commitment to lose weight.

At this juncture, Dr. B decided to go on a water fast. He declared that he would not eat or drink anything except water during the entire period of fasting.

On the other hand, Dr. K decided to go on a fruit fast. He decided that he would eat only fruits and nothing else during the period of fasting.

From that point on, we noticed that Dr. B never came to the cafeteria till the end of his fast. However, Dr. K would come in the cafeteria, pick up some fruit, and leave. He never sat down for dinner with other residents.

The very next day, when I crossed Dr. B, I asked him how it is going. He said, "Good, so far." It is day one. I gave him my thumbs up to show my support. The following day, again as we crossed each other, before I asked him anything, he said, "Day number two. Good so far." And I gave my thumbs up again to show my support. This continued on daily basis to the extent it became a routine.

Although it had become a routine, every day was different. Every day, he had more energy, confidence, and excitement, and he also had a bigger smile and a bigger greeting.

It was a very similar situation with Dr. K. Every time we crossed each other, I showed him my support by giving my thumbs up, and so did many others.

Since it was a community hospital, most resident crossed each other several times a day while making rounds. Every time we crossed each other, we said something positive and encouraging.

Everybody was aware of what was happening—how these two residents had taken the initiative to set an example for themselves. Everybody was trying to cheer them up

This event was extremely important not only in the life of these two residents but also in the history of the hospital.

Both medical residents were so strongly committed and determined that they had absolutely no loss of energy. They were still working their normal schedule from 8:00 a.m. to 11:00 p.m.

This kept on going for twenty-seven days till the end of their fast.

On the twenty-seventh day, i.e., the end of the month of November, one had lost twenty-seven pounds and the other had lost twenty-six pounds. It was decided that both were winners, and nobody had to pay for the other's dinner. Thereafter, we all went for dinner and paid for ourselves, and this is how we all celebrated.

This incident had raised the self-esteem and confidence of both residents, and everybody talked about them. They became the stars of the hospital.

The third resident, who did not participate, felt as if he had lost something. Maybe an opportunity.

Both residents told their stories to every patient who needed to lose weight, for the sole purpose of encouragement. They said if they could do it, anybody can do it. Their statement had a positive impact on many patients, as they were the live examples.

I asked both the residents independently how they felt. Both replied independently, "It was not as hard as we thought initially."

Dr. B also stated that he may do it again in future. "This period of fasting not only made me strong; I also feel that my body is clean and toxic-free, and my mind is sharp. In addition, I have learned the value of fasting."

Dr. B also commented, "Since I fasted, my senses are sharper. My taste buds are stronger, and now I enjoy food much more than I ever did before. Now I can really taste the bread, the milk, the meat, and so on. I also feel lighter every day, and **the best thing that I have learned from this experience is to have control over myself**."

This incident had an effect on many hospital personnel such as nurses, medical staff, and paramedical staff. I also went to the library several times, and each time, I met some people in the library, searching for weight loss information in books or on the Internet. Many people asked the librarian to search for information on this topic.

Because of this wave of interest in weight loss, some of the people also tried to follow the program on a smaller scale and were successful to an extent. Some may have lost couple of pounds, and others more. I also lost a couple of pounds, although I did not have to, nor I was fasting.

This story may also have an impact on you. I am not sure if the phenomenon of weight loss is contagious. (Just kidding.)

A word of caution: During the period of fasting, it is not uncommon to develop a state of euphoria that can lead to fasting too often, and one needs to be aware of that.

A few brief remarks on fasting: Fasting is an extremely common practice among many religious and ethnic groups. It is commonly used to cleanse the body, and strengthen the mind and spirit. Many people do fast in order to prevent diseases and get rid of the toxins from the system. In the natural science of healing, fasting is used as one modality to cure certain medical conditions. Fasting has been in vogue as long as there has been life; however, only recently has fasting developed as a science for the purpose of weight loss.

Story 6

How a Man Beats Cancer and
Pulls Himself from Death's Door

Can you beat cancer?

Kenny says, "Yes!"

On one particular Labor Day weekend, my wife and I were visiting my son in Baltimore, Maryland, when I met Kenny. Although it was one of our regular visits to see our son, this visit became a special one after I met Kenny and heard his very inspiring story. Kenny was the superintendent of the condo complex where my son lived. It was a co-incidence that as soon as we arrived at my son's door, Kenny bumped into us. He introduced himself and asked us if everything is okay. He told us to let him know if we needed anything, and interestingly enough, that led to a long conversation.

A few words about our long weekend trip: My son was doing his surgical residency at John Hopkins University. Although we used to visit him periodically, we barely saw him for half an hour or so even on the long weekend because he was always busy at the hospital. Sometimes he would come home as late as midnight or shortly thereafter, but he always left around 5:00 the next morning. However, that half hour or so with our son was worth the four hours of our one-way trip. Such is the importance of children. This schedule of his used to be quite typical of the most residency programs.

Now, let us return to the story of our new acquaintance Kenny. Here is something about his background:

Kenny is 65 years old, 5'9", weighing 120 pounds. He is the superintendent of an apartment complex. He has a hole in the middle of the front of his neck due to a tracheotomy which he had undergone in the hospital. He can talk and have a good conversation, but he has to block the opening in order to do so. He does that with a handheld device which he carries with him 24/7. He is very optimistic about the whole thing and is proud of his accomplishment.

I asked Kenny, "What happened to you that you have the opening in your neck?"

Thereafter, Kenny started to tell the whole story about the sickness that had changed his life. I think you will appreciate it better if you read Kenny's story in his own words. Thus Kenny continued:

> "Five years ago, I became sick. I was coughing all the time and had difficulty breathing, and this had been going on for more than three months. I was losing weight and had no energy, and I could barely walk, but I was still smoking two packs of cigarettes per day.
> "Although I was very sick, I refused to go to the hospital because I did not like doctors or hospitals. But one morning I started to cough up blood. My wife became nervous and called the ambulance, and they took me to the hospital. They examined me and told me that my lungs were full of blood; therefore, they made a whole in the middle of the neck to insert a tube into my trachea so they could remove the blood from my lungs. They left the tube into my trachea and ran

all kinds of tests in two days. I was told that the procedure that I went through is called tracheostomy.

"The day after all the tests results came back, the doctor in charge came to see me in the morning when my wife and daughter were at my bedside. The doctor had a grim look on his face. I could tell that something was wrong, and my heart started to sink. The doctor sat on my bed and told me that he had bad news for me. I had lung cancer.

"It shocked me and my family, and we were all devastated. The doctor told us a few more things, but we could not understand or remember anything after he told us about the grave diagnosis of lung cancer.

"The following morning, the doctor came again. He further confirmed the diagnosis of lung cancer and told me that my prognosis was bad because the cancer had spread all over my body.

"I asked the doctor, 'What are my chances?'

"The doctor said, 'I am not God, but from my experience, people who are at this stage don't have even 1 percent chance.'

"Next, I asked the doctor, 'How much time do I have?'

"He said, 'Again, I am saying from experience that people who are at your stage have less than three months.'

"Next, I asked the doctor, 'What choices do I have?'

"The doctor replied, 'I can offer you radiation and chemo, but I cannot guarantee anything because your condition is very advanced.'

"Since I had no insurance and no hope, I refused all treatment. My wife and daughter had a big fight with me because they wanted me to go through the treatment. However, I did not listen to anyone and left the hospital against medical advice.

"Back at home, I came to understand that since I had only three months to live, why not enjoy the rest of the time that I have.

"Before going to the hospital, I used to smoke two packs a day, but now I started to smoke even more.

"At this time, I also decided to write a diary about the last days of my life. I went to the store with the intention of buying a diary which had ninety pages because I was told I had only ninety days left, but I could not find one. Therefore, I ended up buying a diary that had one hundred pages. I tore off ten pages. I thought if I had only ninety days to live, I should write something every day for the next ninety days. I was writing everything negative about my life, how I was deteriorating hopelessly, and how life had sucked.

"Besides all of the above, I still continued to smoke three packs a day. I was still drinking Diet Coke and eating all kinds of junk food such as chips and pretzels and so on. This used to be my most favorite diet. I was going from bad to worse every day, but this kept on going for thirty-five days. With each passing day, I was getting weaker and weaker and losing weight. I had no hope in sight or mind.

"After I had spent thirty-five days in misery, something happened. If I look back, I will call it a miracle. It was one Sunday morning. I was sitting in my yard, the weather was beautiful, the birds were flying, and the sun was warm. The flowers were at the peak of their blooming. I heard the ringing of the church bell. Next, I saw a young couple passing by, and they were laughing and giggling. I thought they were on their honeymoon. (I live on a waterfront, and many people come here for their honeymoon.) They said hello to me, smiled, and left.

"All of a sudden a light bulb lit in my head, a spark of hope entered me, and my inside awakened. I became hopeful. I said to myself, 'Kenny, you can sit and rot here for next fifty-five days or you can do something about your condition.' Thereafter in matter of seconds, I made up my mind that I was not going to die. I shall beat death.

"As soon as I made that decision, all of a sudden I got a surge of energy. I do not know where it came from. I felt strong, and I made a commitment to myself that I would beat cancer. At this juncture, I started to recall the stories of the people who had conquered cancer. I began to believe at that time that the mind can do anything, and miracles can happen.

"With all that excitement, I went into the kitchen and told my wife I was not going to die; I would beat cancer. My wife looked at me as if I had gone crazy or something had gone wrong with me or I had lost my mind. She became kind of scared. She watched me closely for next couple of hours, but I knew I was not insane.

"The first thing I did was to throw away all my cigarettes. The next thing I did was to empty my refrigerator of all the junk food that I had stored. I did that in matter of minutes because I was in state of excitement. I also threw away all my junk books which I used to enjoy. Thereafter, I drove to the library in search of cancer cures. I thought I was the only one who could cure cancer because doctors had given me no hope. From that day on, I started to believe in God and miracles, and most importantly, I began to believe in myself.

"On that day, my life took 180° turn and began to transform. I started to go for short walks and then longer walks and then little longer and so on. I started to eat healthy. I changed my diet and started to eat a fair amount of fruits and vegetables. I started to go to church and began reading positive literature, whereas in the past I read junk and sexy books. I felt that my life was changing by the hour, and I was getting better and better every day. And in a matter of next three months, I had so much energy that I was convinced that I no longer had cancer.

"One evening while having dinner with my wife and daughter, I told them in a joking manner that I think that now I am cancer free. The next day, my wife and daughter took me to my doctor for a checkup. My daughter told the doctor, 'Please check my daddy because he believes that he has no cancer.'

"She also told the doctor, 'My father does not smoke, and he eats healthy, including lots of fruits and vegetables. He stopped eating all junk food. Now he also go to the church which he never did before. My daddy is always reading books on how to beat cancer. Now my daddy is gaining weight and is full of his energy, and the color of the face has returned to normal. I also think that my daddy does not have cancer because he looks so healthy.'

"At the request of my daughter, the doctor ran all the tests again. To his amazement, he could not find any evidence of cancer. He thought he had made some mistake in the previous diagnosis. He reviewed all of the previous tests which had showed that I was loaded with cancer. The doctor was amazed and so were I, my wife, and my daughter. She started to cry out of joy, but I took pride in myself, and we all went home.

"Incidentally, this day happened to be my birthday. My daughter and my wife gave me the best birthday party that I ever had in years. I still remember it of this day. They told me, 'This is your new life, and your new birthday.'

"Look, this incident happened five years ago, and I am still alive and in good shape, although I was given only three months to live, and less than 1 percent chance."

Kenny concluded his story with the statement, "A person with strong mind who believes in himself or herself can do anything." (And I think he was right.)

I met Kenny for the second time, ten years after his initial diagnosis of cancer, and he was still alive and cancer free. I had no further contact with Kenny after that date.

At many occasions, I have been faced with the question, "Doctor, can you cure cancer?"

I say, "I cannot, but you may, and few people have done it."

Above is one story of an exceptional person who believed in himself and in the power of his mind. I have heard a few more stories of a similar nature, but this was a real one. I know such stories are not common, but they do exist. I believe as long as there are people who have powerful mind and who believe in themselves, such stories will continue to be reported.

For your information, cancer is a failing of the body and of the immune system due to lack of energy. You may be aware of the fact that cancer is a multi-factorial disease, i.e., there is no single cause that can be attributed to cancer. Cancer attacks us only when our immune system and energy is low.

So, if you can build up your energy and immune system, you may be able to beat cancer. You must have a powerful mind, desire, determination, and the will to live. Doctors and medicine cannot do that for you, but you may be able to do it.

In my fifty years of medical practice, I have learned a lot of lessons, and this was one of the good ones. This story made me think that even if there is 1 percent chance of surviving any illness, who knows this may be my lucky patient.

You all know that the man as a whole is more powerful than his disease or condition, and an awakened person can do wonders.

I would like to say a few words about statistics before concluding this chapter. Statistics is a science where people put numbers on graph or tabular form. I want to tell you very clearly and emphatically that statistics applies to a group but not to an individual.

Let me clarify that point by two examples:

Take the example of Kenny. He was given less than 1 percent chance and less than ninety days to live, but he made it with flying colors.

So, if a person makes it, how does it matter if his chances were 1 percent or 99 percent? To Kenny, the chance of less than 1 percent turned out to be 100 percent as far as he was concerned.

Let us take a reverse scenario. A patient is suffering from a not-so-serious disease, but the chance of dying from that disease is only 1 percent. If the patient dies because he falls in that unlucky 1 percent, as far as that patient is concerned, disease is 100 percent fatal.

This should be a big lesson for you or anyone.

Some people say where there is a will, there is hope, and I have to agree with that.

I believe as long as there are people like Kenny, we shall continue to read or hear similar stories in the future.

Story 7

The Best Peanut Ever

Have you ever had the opportunity to meet a swami (spiritual master) of the highest caliber? If you did, you must know how rewarding and awesome that experience can be. This story is about such a personal experience.

One day around 2:00 p.m. in the hot month of July, my father and I entered the cottage of a swami. As we entered the cottage, Swamiji was giving a discourse. Approximately ten people were sitting there, and two of them were teenagers. It was obvious from the behavior of the teenagers that they were not interested in being there; they were looking here and there. It appeared that they were made to come. I could understand their feeling because I was also a teenager; however, I used to go with my father because I enjoyed his company.

As soon as we entered the cottage, we noticed that Swamiji was sitting on a raised platform so that everybody could see him. We bowed our heads to Swamiji, and he gave his blessing by raising his right hand. (This is typically that swamis do.)

Next, my father offered some fruit to Swamiji, and this is called the offering or Dakshna. There is also a place by the side of a swami where one can place the offering.

When you visit a swami, you generally do not go empty-handed. Most people bring some kind of offering; some bring fruits, others bring nuts, and some offer money, and so on. It is out of honor or respect, not a tuition or fee that you have to give. However, many people do so because they believe that if they want to get something worthwhile, they must pay something for it, otherwise they may not get the benefit. Anyhow, after giving the offering, we also sat on the floor like everyone else.

Swamiji was in his mid-fifties, calm with a kind look about him. His face was red and head shiny. He spoke in a assuring and the sweet language. You could feel that he was a caring person and also quite advanced in his spiritual accomplishment.

The atmosphere of the cottage was very serene. There was a special aroma there which had kind of a cooling nature. It was just perfect for the hot month of July. You could also hear the murmuring of a spring nearby. On that day, it had just rained, so the wind was not as dry and piercing but moist. It felt good.

While Swamiji was giving the discourse, one of his servants offered water to everyone. This was also a typical routine in India because most visitors come from hot climates and are thirsty.

After half an hour or so, the same servant brought some peanuts in small individual containers for everyone, including one for Swamiji.

In the discourse, Swamiji was talking about his experience and how he became a swami. The one-hour discourse was very interesting. I observed that during the discourse, every now and then he would pick up a peanut and put it into his mouth. It looked as if he was not interested in the peanuts or in a hurry to eat them.

He had not finished his peanuts even by the end of his discourse, but I ate my peanuts in five minutes, and it might have taken little longer for my father to finish his.

I can tell you that these peanuts were warm, well roasted, and smelled great. **These were the best peanuts I had ever eaten.**

Now, coming back to the discourse, Swamiji stated that he came from a Brahmin family. The Brahmin caste is a respectable caste amongst Hindus and can be compared to a priest's family. Swamiji said that his father was very obese as he used to overeat. This was kind of a requirement of their profession; people do over-feed Brahmins for their own personal benefit.

"As the result of obesity, my father had developed high blood pressure, diabetes, and high cholesterol. He also had lost one leg as a result of diabetes, and later on he developed heart disease." Swamiji said that his father died at the age of fifty-seven of a heart attack.

Swamiji continued, "The death of my father and his diabetes brought an awakening in my life, and I had made up my mind that I would lose weight so that I never have to go through this problem in my life. I also used to be obese and had a touch of diabetes, as well as a problem with blood pressure. My doctor had been telling me in the past to lose weight, but I had ignored his advice till that date, but now things changed. Now I eat only if I need to, not because I want to. Now I do not eat for the sake of enjoyment but out of necessity. I told myself that food is not fun; the only purpose of food is health. As a result, I lost a lot of weight, and as I was losing weight, my medical condition gradually disappeared. Now I am of the right weight for my height, and I have no diseases, and my mental clarity has improved a lot. Now I realize how bad and dangerous obesity can be."

Swamiji stressed that we human beings need to focus on the mission or goal of life and not on food. We should eat to live and not live to eat. Both the quality and the quantity of food have an affect not only our body but also on the mind.

My father asked him, "Swamiji, you have mentioned that people over-feed Brahmins. Why so?"

Swamiji replied, "Because there are some Hindus who believe that whatever food goes into the stomach of a Brahmin, it will also go into the stomach of their dead ancestors, and the dead ancestors will be pleased. Such is the extent of belief. So, people over-feed Brahmins to keep their ancestors happy. These Hindus invite Brahmins after the death of a dear one. Some people even invite Brahmins years after year on the death anniversary."

One gentleman asked, "Swamiji, why did it take you so long to finish your peanuts?"

Swamiji replied, "The more slowly you eat, the more likely you will enjoy the food and the more benefit you will derive from the food. Also when you enjoy more, you are more likely to eat less."

Swamiji also stressed one very interesting point, "When you eat slowly, it is more likely you will be more content in life." He mentioned that each grain of food is loaded with energy, and in reality we do not need much food to survive. Can you imagine that from one peanut or seed, you can grow a plant?

Next, we stood up and bowed our heads. Swamiji gave his blessing by raising his right hand, and then we left for home.

Let me give you some interesting background as to how we ended up in the cottage of the Swamiji.

The city where Swamiji lived is known as Rishi Kesh. This is a special town where many spiritual masters live; the words Rishi Kesh literally means residence of swamis or spiritual masters. This has been one of my father's most favorite places for vacation because he had a keen interest in spiritual knowledge and was in his search of a spiritual master. To fulfill this desire or quest and to meet spiritual masters, he had a routine to close his business for one week every year in July when we children were all off from school.

In his search for a spiritual master, he would go from one cottage to another and try to meet as many swamis as possible. Typically, he will visit a swami, sit there for a while, listen to the discourse or will have conversation with the master, and if he enjoyed that, he would spend hours and hours there and even revisit him. Otherwise, he would leave after a short while.

The remainder of the family also enjoyed their vacation or had fun in their own way. Some loved to eat and sleep, others had fun with games, some enjoyed rich food and afternoon naps, some enjoyed swimming, and still others went for long walks, and so on.

Rishi Kesh is a holy, spiritual and, is quite an interesting city, a suburb of another city named Hardwar. In order to go to Rishi Kesh, we had to go through the city of Hardwar, a big city with a large population and a great transportation system, whereas the city of Rishi Kesh is a small town only a couple of miles away from this city. Both cities are connected with each other with bus or taxi. There is no train system for Rishi Kesh. However, both cities are considered spiritual, and both are located on the banks of Ganges River.

Hardwar is extremely important and popular for many reasons. Firstly, it is also a place where many Swamiji or spiritual masters lived, just like Rishi Kesh. Secondly, it is a place where most Hindus go for the final rites of their dear ones. Since this city is located at the banks of the Ganges River and has facilities for taking baths, this adds to its importance because some Hindus believe that taking a bath in this river washes away their sins, and therefore Hindus go there year after year to take a bath in this river and to wash away their sins. Such is the perception of some people; however, the reality and perception at times becomes difficult to differentiate.

As far as city of Rishi Kesh is concerned, it is a beautiful and awesome place. The moment you enter the city, you feel like you are in heaven. The soothing sound of Ganges River, the large grass fields, the open spaces, the fruit-laden trees, the flowers, and the chirping of the birds overtake you and make you forget everything, even the pain and misery of daily life at the least for those moments. Even during July, somehow you do not feel that hot because the atmosphere is so serene. You wish that you could stay there forever.

Now, coming back to the meeting with Swamiji, after having this great experience with him, we left for home on foot. It was approximately a one-mile walk. My father also narrated couple of more interesting stories about other spiritual masters on our way home. My father was a good storyteller, and I believe this was his way of educating me.

As soon as we reached home, my mother was waiting for us. She asked where we had gone. My father said, "Today we had a very interesting experience meeting with a swami." My mother became curious and next my father called every family member to come and listen to the story of our meeting with Swamiji.

My father stressed that Swamiji had told us that eating slowly has multiple benefits. Eating slowly and chewing food well aids digestion and prevents overeating, thereby helping keep normal weight. "As you know, overeating can lead to obesity and multiple problems associated with it such as diabetes, hypertension, and cholesterol issues," he said. He also stressed that people who eat their food slowly are more content in their lives.

My father also said, "Swamiji told us that we do not need much food because each grain is loaded with energy."

After hearing this story, my mother said to all of us, "Look, I had been telling you all along that you should take your time to eat, chew your food well, and do not rush. In that way, you will digest your food more easily.

Thereafter, we had our delicious dinner, and everybody went to sleep. However, I kept thinking about the meeting with Swamiji, the delicious and warm peanuts, and the story that my father told me on our way to home. I kept thinking about what Swamiji had said repeatedly: if we eat slowly, we will be also more content in life. Somehow this did not make any sense to me at that time, but now it surely does.

I also observed that from that day on, everybody ate slowly and a little less food than they were used to eating. As a result, a couple of my family members, who had been obese, lost weight. I also noticed that one of our family members who had some tense temperament became little calmer in his nature. I used to think that it may have been due to his eating more slowly.

I cannot imagine how a little story like this could bring a change in the behavior of my family members, and it may also affect yours.

The behavior and the habits of a person can make or break his or her physical and mental health.

Story 8

Just a Cup of Tea

What can you expect from the cup of tea?

I have been very fortunate to have had the opportunity to meet and converse with several spiritual masters in my life, and all of them had something to offer. For example, one master taught me how to increase concentration, other taught me how to control my breath, and yet another taught me how to improve my digestion. In the previous story, we learned that by eating slowly, we can increase our contentment level.

Here is my story of meeting with another great spiritual master:

During one very hot day in July, my father and I entered the cottage of a spiritual master at approximately 5:30 p.m. My father did not know him, but that was quite typical. People come and go as they please, and anyone is welcome there. People who come are those who want to have a spiritual touch, but for some it is a yearly routine. When we entered the cottage, we noticed that the master was sitting in the Lotus position with his eyes closed, and there was nobody else there at that time, so we just sat down.

Swamiji must have been in his late sixties or early seventies. He wore clothes typical of a swami, a mixture of red and yellow, which typically is a saffron color and quite popular among swamis.

The whole atmosphere was calm and serene in the cottage. Occasionally, we could hear the chirping of birds and the soothing sound of a fountain nearby, and we could feel the breeze at times.

We felt the freshness, the energy, and cleanliness of the air. The cottage was filled with the beautiful aroma of roses.

We waited for the master to open his eyes, so my father could have a conversation with him. My father used to enjoy this kind of opportunity and meeting. We waited for a very long time, but Swamiji neither moved nor blinked his eyes; he was like a statue. After a long wait, I became kind of impatient, but my father did not. I must have been thirteen years of age at that time, and I did not have the patience to wait for that long, and I wasn't interested in the spiritual conversation. It was the different story for my father. The longer the Swamiji kept his eyes closed or did not move, the more curious and determined my father became, just to have a conversation with him. My father used to say that the longer a swami stays in Samadhi (focused concentration), the more accomplished he is, the more one should be able to learn from him.

As I became impatient every few minutes, I would touch my father and ask him how much longer we had to wait. My father would say just a little longer, and this kept going on for a while. I kept asking how much longer, and my father kept repeating his favorite answer: just a little longer. Once I realized that my father was determined to have a conversation with the master, I became quiet and accepted the fact that I had no choice but to wait.

In one and a half hour, while we were waiting, many people came and went. Some stayed for fifteen minutes, others for half an hour. Nobody was as determined as my father, nor did anybody have the patience of my father.

After a long wait, finally the Swamiji opened his eyes, and I breathed a sigh of relief. We bowed our heads in his honor, and he blessed us by raising his right hand. Then my father started to have a conversation with him. At that time, Swamiji ordered water for all of us and three cups of tea, one for himself and two for us.

First, we drank the cold water which was much needed because of the very hot weather, and thereafter we drank our tea. My father and I drank our tea in a matter of several minutes, but Swamiji continued to sip that cup of tea for half an hour as long as we were having a conversation with him.

At the end of discourse, it was already 7:30 p.m. At this juncture, Swamiji asked my father if we would stay for the dinner. This was just a courteous question from the spiritual master. If you visit a swami during the meal time, he will ask you that question. Fortunately, my father said no. I thanked God over and over again. I was thinking that if it took half an hour for Swamiji to drink a cup of tea, how long would it take for him to eat his dinner? I was also thinking that if my father said yes for dinner, I might have been stuck there for the whole night.

Next, Swamiji called his servant and told him that he would not take his dinner as he felt satisfied with the delicious cup of tea that was very fulfilling.

Now my father became more curious and asked Swamiji, "How could you live on just a cup of tea?"

The master replied, "Spiritual people are more aware of their body, mind, and soul, and have better control on their lives. Spiritual people know that you do not need much food to live on. Some spiritual masters can even live on air." Then he narrated the story of a swami who never eats. He told the story of a saint who never sleeps, and so on. He further stressed the point that it is all in the power of the mind. I do not remember the whole conversation that my father had with Swamiji, but I could not get over the fact that anybody could live without food or on just a cup of tea. This was beyond comprehension for a teenager, but I knew that Swamis always tell the truth, and later on I confirmed the validity of this fact from spiritual literature.

Swamiji also told my father that the more food we eat, the more desire and discontentment there will be. He stressed that overeating beyond our needs can cause health problems such as diabetes high blood pressure, cholesterol issues, etc., and it can also reduce our life expectancy.

Swamiji continued, "In the materialistic world, people look at what is out there for them, but in the spiritual world, we focus on what is within us. We have everything within us and we are our own source of energy. We need to understand the power of the mind, and that we are the perfect creation of God."

Next, my father gave his offering as a token of appreciation. We bowed our heads again in honor, and Swamiji blessed us again by raising his right hand before we left.

When we got home, everybody was waiting for us for dinner.

Before dinner, my father shared the experience of our meeting with Swamiji with the whole family, and the fact that the swami's dinner was just a cup of tea.

After hearing this story, my mother was taken a little aback and became quiet because she had a tendency to overfeed us, although she used to tell us that we must eat slowly and chew the food well.

Thereafter, my mother served the dinner to all of us. However, I noticed this day was a different from other days. Everybody ate a little less than usual, and there was more calmness at the table.

On that night before going to bed, I kept wondering how people can live on little or no food, and, more importantly, how this little story affected my family members.

Ever since this incident, I have been observing difference between the habits and behavior of healthy versus overweight people. The healthy people choose their food carefully, eat slowly, and are more content in life.

There are many levels of Swamis or spiritual masters. Some are just beginners, but a majority of them are in the middle. There are only a very few who are at the peak of their accomplishment. It is always good to know the level of the spiritual master with whom you are having a conversation.

Story 9

The Fish Oil Cure for Arthritis

One Wednesday morning, I was sitting in my office trying to catch up with my paperwork, and that was a typical day of for me. All of a sudden, I was interrupted by a phone call from the owner of a company for which I was the company doctor. He told me that something has flown into his right eye, and he needed to come over and have me take this thing out of his eye. Since I was his company doctor, I could not say no.

I removed the foreign body from his eye. Thereafter, we had a one-hour conversation, and it turned out to be interesting and productive. I enjoyed that meeting. I have always been impressed with this gentleman because he is a very caring person who treats his employees extremely well, just like family members. According to my observation, this is not common these days. I can cite some incidents that I have witnessed myself to support this statement:

I used to go to his company every year in October to give flu shots to all of his employees, and every one had to stand in a line to get their shot. To my surprise, he also stood in the same line as everyone else and joked with them. I was very impressed with his friendly behavior.

I made another observation. I used to treat his employees if and when they got injured at work. What I noticed was that the employee wanted to go back to work after the treatment of their injury. However, my experience had been quite different when I treated employees from other companies; they invariably asked me to give them a day or two off.

I shall cite you one more incident: Once I had the opportunity to visit his company personally for some reason, and I was impressed with the friendly atmosphere that prevailed there. I believe this was at least one of the reasons that his company was flourishing while most companies were wrapping up their business because of the bad economy.

Now, let's go back to my one-hour conversation with this employer. During our talk, he asked me a question, "How do I treat arthritis?"

I told him I have several ways to treat arthritis. "I can give conventional medicine such as a painkiller and/or prescribe a non-steroidal medication such as ibuprofen. And if a person is overweight, I always tell them to lose weight because I have observed that even a loss of ten to fifteen pounds can make a difference in the arthritic condition. In many cases, where it is the beginning of arthritis, I have prescribed Chondroitin with Glucosamine with success, and many cases I treat homeopathically. I can also prescribe a diet based upon Ayurvedic principles or on the principles of the acid and alkaline nature of the food, so on and so forth."

Then I asked him, "Why did you ask me this question? Do you have a problem with arthritis?"

He asked, "Have you heard of the fish oil cure for arthritis?"

I said, "No, please tell me about it."

This is what he said:

> "I used to suffer from very bad arthritis of the knees, hips, and hands," he said. "I tried all kinds of medicines that had side effects. I did not know what to choose: the pain of arthritis or the side effects of the medications. I also became aware of the fact that the treatment of arthritis is not that simple just because of the side effects of the medication used. So I decided that I have to find a cure for my condition myself because medication was not the answer. Thereafter, I started to investigate the natural cures for arthritis. Finally I found a book on the fish oil cure for arthritis. Next, I decided to give it a try, and it worked. I have told many of my friends of this cure. They are all happy about it."

I asked him, "Can you tell me little more about your fish oil cure?"

"You should take one teaspoon of fish oil from cold water fish, mix it with four ounces of orange juice, shake it vigorously, and then drink on an empty stomach and then not eat anything for half an hour."

At this juncture, I asked him to please explain in little more detail so that I could experiment with it.

He continued:

> 1. Fish oil has to be liquid form and not in capsules.

> 2. Fish oil has to be from cold water fish such as from Alaska, United Kingdom, etc., and not fish from warm climate like Florida or Texas.

3. The orange juice should be fresh, preferably.

4. You must shake it vigorously so that the fish oil disappears in the juice.

5. You must drink it on an empty stomach.

6. You should not eat or drink anything for at least half an hour.

I asked him about the rationale of this treatment. He said, "When fish oil is taken this way, it does not get digested, but it goes directly into the joints and becomes part of the lubricant, and also it has anti-inflammatory properties."

After finishing my day at the office, I went to the library and got the book that he has recommended. I read the book from the beginning to the end and was quite impressed with the fish oil cure. I cannot remember the author or the title of the book because this incident happened close to twenty-five years ago.

My experience with the fish oil cure for the arthritis has been rewarding. I started using this formula for the patients who have been suffering from arthritis. It did not matter whether they had arthritis of the knee, hip, shoulder, or any other joint.

However, the degree of benefit that people got varied from patient to patient. People with mild arthritis got the maximum benefits; however, people with moderate or severe arthritis were also able to get only some benefit. Anyhow, most patients were able to reduce their pain medication to some degree or the other, and in some cases, it was quite significant.

There are several types of arthritis—osteoarthritis, rheumatoid arthritis, gout, and so on. One of the key elements to differentiate arthritis types one from the other is if it is inflammatory by nature.

The fish oil cure has been used mostly for osteoarthritis, which is non-inflammatory and more or less a degenerative disease. The formula has not been studied with inflammatory arthritis.

My new experience: One day, a patient came to me who was in his late fifties and had been suffering from rheumatoid arthritis, a condition that is inflammatory. He asked me, "Do you have a natural cure for my condition?

I told him I had been trying this formula for osteoarthritis but not for his condition. He told me he would give it try because he would not take any conventional medicine because of their side effects. He told me that he had tried many medicines, but they all have side effects. Some medications have a negative effect on the kidneys, others on the liver, and even one has a negative effect on the eyes.

I saw this patient after a year for something else. I asked him if he had tried the fish oil cure. He said he has been using that formula ever since and felt much better. He further stated that now he can get by without pain medication with the exception of Tylenol. He said he was very pleased with this formula, although he is not 100 percent better.

If you ask my opinion, I cannot say this formula alone is a cure for every kind of arthritis, but I would say that this formula makes an important contribution to the arthritis cure.

If you ask me if it is worth a try, I would say emphatically, yes.

One more fact readers should know is that eating an alkaline diet could also help arthritis to a great degree because acidity is one of the important contributing factors to arthritis, as well as many other diseases.

You might be aware of the fact that there is an abundance of literature on the subject of acid and alkaline diet. I have also observed that the diet based upon the Ayurvedic principles, also reduces the inflammation and pain of the arthritis, as it balances the dosha. I also have addressed this issue in my previous book.

Story 10

Unique Patient – Unique Ways

One Monday morning 8:00, a regular patient of mine called and said that she needed to see me immediately because she was desperate. I gave her an early appointment at that hour, even before I started the office.

On entering the examining room, I said, "Hi, Patty. How are you?"

Patty replied, "Dr. Singhal, I hate myself. I look ugly. I had a fight with my husband the other night, and he yelled at me, and in a way he was right. I need to do something about my weight and smoking.

I asked her to tell me more about what had happened and why she was so upset.

Patty continued:

> "Yesterday was Sunday, and I was off from work. I woke up late in the morning and was very relaxed. My husband had taken my children to a game, and I was at home alone. I was ready to take a shower when I saw myself nude in front of the whole body mirror. It shocked me, and I could not believe myself, how ugly I look. I felt as though I have never looked at myself like this before.
>
> "It was the first time that I noticed that my belly is hanging halfway to the knees, and my neck is getting fat and shorter. Now people cannot even see my thyroid gland in my neck. My thighs are bumpy, and I have ugly legs. It was also the first time that I came to the realization that I had been getting short of breath

whenever I go up the steps. I had been noticing recently that when I tried to tie my shoelaces, my belly got in the way. I must lose weight now and get into shape. I cannot afford to look like this. I feel ugly. Dr. Singhal, I am ready to do anything. It was a wake-up call for me."

She cried a bit and then continued,

"I feel as if there must be a mistake on my part. Why had I been ignoring the advice of my doctor, the nagging comments of my children, and the look of my husband who had been telling me do something about my weight? They were all saying to me indirectly that I must lose weight.

"To make matters worse, the other night my husband had a big fight with me. He told me that I must quit smoking at least if I did not want to do anything about my weight. 'You are also exposing all of us to the secondhand smoke and our children do not deserve that,' he said. 'From now on, if you have to smoke, at least go out of the house.' My husband was right. I must quit smoking. As a matter of fact, I do not like smoking at all. But I'm afraid that if I quit smoking, I will gain weight and blow up like a balloon, and that is the only reason I smoke."

I said, "Patty, I do understand your situation. Tell me where do you want me to start?"

"I think the best thing for me is to stop smoking, but I'm scared that I will gain weight."

"Patty, from experience, I can tell you that after most patients stop smoking, they do not gain weight, although some may do. It all depends on the individual. You have to have a mindset and then you will not gain weight."

"Are you sure I will not gain weight?" she pleaded.

I told her, "Yes, you will not gain weight if you do not want to, as I have just explained to you."

Next I examined Patty. She is 43 years old, 5'2," and weighs 265 pounds. Her blood pressure is 120/80. She does not drink alcohol. However, she smokes one pack a day and has been smoking for twenty-five years. She had no surgeries in the past and does not have any other medical condition. She is happily married and has two children. She has been patient of mine for almost nine years. She is a nurse at the nearby hospital.

After examination, I told her to come back in five days for her next appointment.

She came back after five days for her scheduled appointment for my stop-smoking program. I administered the one-hour program, and, as a result, she quit smoking. I followed her for two weeks, and she did not gain any weight. She had not smoked, and now I was convinced of the power of hypnosis.

Two weeks later, she came back for help with weight loss. I took a detailed history as to the cause of her obesity. She told me something very interesting. "I never sit down to eat a healthy meal, but I snack all day long, and on the wrong foods. I got this habit from my mother. I never saw her eating a good meal. She was always snacking, although she always fed us healthy meals."

Next, I told Patty that her role as a mother in bringing up her children is extremely important, and she needed to set an example for them. I advised that children typically follow what parents do, just like she had followed her mother's lifestyle. Thereafter, I educated her about the importance of healthy diet, and that snacking here and there usually ends up not being healthy, and also eating too much contributes to weight gain.

In our next session, I hypnotized her for weight loss and followed her closely. She did fairly well under the circumstances. I am not providing the detail of the program as it has been discussed in the previous stories. In short, I advised her to cut down on the portion size of her meals, to eat plenty of vegetables and fruits, to exercise regularly and, most importantly, to have a positive mindset.

I followed her for two more sessions and she had made good progress and was pleased with it.

What intrigued me was that she had been looking herself in the same mirror for many years. What was so different that one day than all of the other days before it?

What I have been noticing as a physician is that everybody has his or her own triggers. When the time for change comes, things start to change and mold. Just take the case of Patty. It was hard to predict what triggered the change: a fight with her husband or just the right time for a change or the right time for an awakening.

At times, this is how things work in life!

Many people are unique, and so are their ways.

Story 11

The Lady Who Lived in a Coke Bottle

Do you think a lady can live in a Coke bottle?

One afternoon, Kathy came to me with the following complaints:

1. Abdominal distention for six months

2. Pain in both knees for nine months

Kathy is 27 years old, 4' 11" and 215 pounds. She does not smoke or drink. She takes only Advil for joint pain and Pepcid for acidity, but at times she takes Tums instead of Pepcid. She further states that every now and then, she uses her asthma pump. She denies any history of diabetes, high blood pressure or cholesterol, and had had no surgery in the past. She is a housewife and mother of three children.

On further inquiry, she told me that on many occasions, her belly becomes very much distended, and she belches a lot of gas, and passes flatus from below. She says at times her abdomen gets so big that she has difficulty breathing and has to use the asthma pump. She also states that she gets heartburn quite often.

Regarding her knee pain, it started nine months ago and has been getting progressively worse. She states that her knee hurts only when she walks but not if she's sitting at rest.

She admits that she is addicted to Coke. She starts her day with Coke and ends her day with Coke, and of course she drinks Coke all day long. She loves Coke so much that if she does not get

Coke, she gets nervous and agitated. She told me that she got this Coke habit from her parents. Both parents used to drink Coke, and both were obese and diabetic. She also admitted that at times she lets her children drink Coke because she thinks it is good for digestion.

One time, her husband told me separately in confidence that his wife was addicted to Coke. There is a Coke everywhere in the house, and the house smells like Coke. There is a Coke in the bedroom, TV room, kitchen, and even in the car. She also keeps an icebox in the car where she always keeps a few cans of Coke.

After taking her history, I gave her a full physical. Then I tested her blood for diabetes, liver, kidney, thyroid, and also for arthritis. All tests came out negative. Examination of the knees was also normal. Thereafter, I sent her for x-rays of the knees, and they were also normal.

Then I explained to her that in my opinion her condition was due to the acidity of Coke. Acidity not only affects the stomach but also the calcium metabolism that affects bones and joints.

She replied in resentment, "How that could be? I have been drinking Coke all my life. Why is it affecting me now?"

"Now you are twenty-seven years old," I explained, "and the Coke has caught up to you."

Then she told me that her sister is thirty-five years old, and she drinks even more Coke but has no problems.

I explained to her that everybody is different, and everybody reacts differently, and she should not compare herself with her sister.

Next I asked her, "Do you like milk?"

"I hate it," she said, making faces

Next I asked her, "Do you like vegetables such as broccoli, carrots, cucumbers, cauliflower, and so on?"

She replied that she hates vegetables.

I explained to her that she needed to stop drinking Coke and start taking calcium tablets. This would help her stomach and joint problems.

She told me she would take calcium tablets, but she cannot do without Coke.

Then I suggested that she drink Coke-flavored water. She replied that is not possible.

After a tough negotiation, I made her agree that she would drink water and Coke mixture in the ratio of nine parts of water and one part of Coke.

I noticed that during this conversation, her husband kept quiet. Whenever I looked at him, he will turn away his face. I got the impression that he did not want to say anything. Most likely, he wanted to avoid any arguments or fights at a later date. Whenever I told her to stop drinking Coke to help her condition, her husband nodded in agreement with me, although he did not speak a word.

I saw Kathy again six weeks later. She had a little smile on her face. She told me her knee pain was all gone and her stomach was at least 50 percent better. Her belly does not get distended, but she still gets little heartburn now and then, but overall she feels much better.

On this visit, she made the following remarks: "Today for the first time, I'm convinced how bad the Coke can be. I never would have guessed that in a million years. Thank you for bringing that awakening in me. I know at times I have been resentful of your suggestions, and I feel sorry for that. Now I have made up my mind that I will not let Coke enter in my home because of what I have been through."

I congratulated her about her achievement of not drinking Coke. I told her to see me back in two months and to continue the same treatment.

On her last visit, she told me that she had not touched Coke ever since. " I am now hundred percent convinced that Coke was the cause of all my problems." She also told me that ever since her last visit, she had not used her asthma pump.

I needed to see her only three times for her condition.

You may want to know that an acidic body is the cause of multiple diseases and problems, whereas an alkaline body is the basis of health. Going little further, one also needs to know that it is acidic food that makes the body acidic, and conversely, alkaline food makes an alkaline healthy body.

For your information, Coke is one of the most acidic beverages. Other acidic foods are: meats, desserts, alcoholic beverages, pickles, teas, and coffee. Fruits and vegetables are the most alkaline foods.

For those of you who want to explore further the subject of acidity and alkalinity, remember there is an abundance of literature on this subject. You can search on the Internet, or go to a library for any of several books on this subject. I have also addressed this subject more thoroughly in my previous book.

Story 12

Professor Johnson and His Diabetes

Here is the story of a professor who has been a patient of mine for the last nine years. He is fifty-seven years old, 5'8" and weighs 253 pounds. His blood pressure is 150/100. He was a smoker for about thirty-five years but quit smoking ten years ago. He drinks alcohol only socially. He never had a physical in the past and therefore was never diagnosed of any medical condition. He is married and has no children, and his wife is a homemaker and does not go to work.

The professor teaches math at the university. He has been so successful that he was able to get his tenure after eight years of being a professor, which some people may not get even after ten years.

Although the professor has been my patient for approximately nine years—an infrequent visitor to the office—he comes in only when he has some acute sickness such as a cold, flu or bronchitis, diarrhea, etc.

For a long time, I have been stressing upon him the importance of a routine physical, but he kept saying someday. At another occasion, he would say, "I feel fine." Once, I was able to convince him to make an appointment for the physical, but he ended up canceling at the last minute. It is hard to understand why he does not want physical; perhaps he does not want to find out what's wrong with him (as is the case with many) or he is too busy for the physical.

One day, he came to me, complaining of chest pain and stated that he wanted to have a good physical. He was scared, had an anxious look, and kept looking into my eyes. He said, "I'm afraid of heart attacks because they run in my family. I know I have been ignoring your advice in the past, but this chest pain is a wake-up call for me. Today, I promise myself in front of you that from now on I shall take care of myself.

Here is his family history: The professor told me that his father had diabetes and, due to his condition, lost one leg. He further added that ten years later, his father's kidneys failed, and he was put on kidney dialysis. It was painful to see his father suffer as a dialysis patient. On the day of his dialysis, he used to be very sick and weak. The professor further told me that his father died of heart attack at the age of sixty-two.

Next, I asked the professor, "Please tell me more about yourself."

He replied:

> "I am married and I have no children. As you know life is very different without children. My wife does not work, and she stays home and has no hobbies. She does not like to cook or shop, and she has no concept of nutrition. She is very fond of doughnuts, and unfortunately, there is a doughnut shop around the corner. Whenever she gets hungry, she takes a ride in her car and buys doughnuts. She eats whatever she likes and then leaves the rest for me. When I go home,

I never get healthy meals unless we go out. I never learned to exercise because my father was not into it, and I cannot blame him for that because I am also kind of lazy."

I gave him a complete physical, took blood, and gave him an EKG. His EKG showed that he has a coronary ischemia. His blood tests showed cholesterol of 300, and his blood glucose at 296. His hemoglobin A-1 C was 8.4, and his serum creatinine was 1.2, which is high for his age. Next, I went over these findings with him, and after a lengthy discussion, I gave him prescriptions for his diabetes and high blood pressure. I also made the following recommendations, based upon the evaluation:

1. He must lose weight. Ideally, he should weigh 170 pounds, however even if he will lose 20 pounds, it can improve his health a great deal. If he continues to lose even one pound per week, he could end up losing 52 pounds in a year.

2. I gave him six hours of diabetic education by the diabetic nurse practitioner. That included understanding his new medical condition, how to test his blood glucose, and how to keep a log of it. In addition, he received information about nutrition, especially in reference to his diabetic condition.

3. I advised him to exercise. When he told me that he has no time, I offered that he could walk to work since he lives on the university campus.

4. I also advised him to eat at least five to six servings of vegetables. When he told me his wife doesn't cook, I told him that most vegetables do not require cooking. For example broccoli, carrots, tomatoes, lettuce,

cucumbers, radishes, and others can be eaten raw, and they taste delicious with dressing; also raw vegetable have added health benefits.

5. I advised him to consume eggs, milk, or cheese for protein. He can also have roasted soya beans or any other beans for his proteins, which do not require any cooking. He was also advised to stop eating donuts.

6. I gave him a prescription for his diabetes and high blood pressure.

I further advised him to see me every two weeks until his conditions became stabilized.

From there on, I saw a complete turnaround in his attitude.

He started to visit me regularly. He kept a log of his blood sugar and blood pressure, and they were all coming down gradually.

After six months, he underwent another physical. His EKG was normal. A stress test was also normal.

He had lost almost thirty-three pounds. His blood pressure had become normal, so I took him off his blood pressure medication, but he still takes medication for his diabetes. He never required insulin injections for which he was very grateful.

This story teaches us one thing: No matter how educated a person may be, everyone is subjected to the same ills and suffering. This story affirms my strong belief that by making changes in one's behavior and adopting a healthy lifestyle, many diseases can be reversed at any age.

Story 13

Doctor, I Have Run Out of Options

Here is an interesting and educational story. Mr. Smith came to my office one Tuesday morning with a persistent cough and shortness of breath. This was his fourth visit this year.

Mr. Smith is 59 years old, 5'9" and weighs 245 pounds. His blood pressure is 160/90, and pulse is 76. His respiration is 18 per minute. He does not smoke or drink and denies having any allergies. He does not take any medications on a regular basis and had no surgeries in the past. He further stated that he had not had a physical in last thirty years. He is married and has two children. He is the owner of a 7-Up store.

After examination, I told Mr. Smith, "Look, you have bronchitis, asthma, and high blood pressure. You are quite overweight and that has lot to do with your condition. This is your fourth visit this year for the same condition. It is time for a good physical, so that I can evaluate your overall health."

He replied in his typical tone and language, "Doctor, I am busy; maybe next time. For now, just give me the prescription for my condition as you always do, and someday you can give me the physical. (He is a typical businessman, either busy or too busy for his physical or anything else that does not give immediate results.)

Two days later, he came back and said, "Dr. Singhal, you're right. I need to lose weight. I think my weight is interfering with my breathing. Today you can prescribe your diet program and then

I will make plans for the physical."

I was surprised to see the complete turnaround in his attitude, and I gave the following program in nutshell:

1. Cut down on the portion size of the meals.

2. Stop snacking in between meals.

3. Cut down on meat portions because they're very concentrated and rich in calories and fat.

4. Exercise half an hour a day, five days a week.

5. Eat plenty for water-rich food, especially vegetables.

He said, "No way! I'm not a saint, and I want to enjoy meat in my life. Can you prescribe diet pills for me?"

I told him, "I cannot recommend that because they will raise your blood pressure, which is already high."

Next he asked me can he go for liposuction.

I told him, "I do not recommend that either as it will not solve the root cause of your problem, but that is your choice. Until you adopt a healthy lifestyle, you cannot expect any permanent result."

I saw him again after four months for another attack of asthma. He had gained another ten pounds. I treated him for the asthma and told him that he should sincerely consider losing weight. He said, "Yes, Dr. Singhal, I agree with you that I must lose weight."

I was again surprised to hear these words from him. I asked him what made him change his mind. He told me that he went to a surgeon for liposuction, but the surgeon wanted to charge him $5,000, and he cannot afford that. The surgeon has also told him that the surgery would not solve the root cause of his problem.

Once again, after noticing a change in his attitude and a desire to work on weight loss program, I discussed the same weight loss program that I had offered him initially.

I saw him two months later, and he has gained another ten pound. I asked him, "Are you following the program?" He said, "I have tried this program, but it is too hard. Therefore I am trying to find another surgeon for liposuction who will charge me less."

When I saw him five months later, he had lost close to thirty-five pounds. I asked him how he had done that. I also asked him if he had gone to the new surgeon.

He started to laugh and then said:

> "Yes, Doctor, I did go to a new surgeon, and he told me that he would charge him only $2,500 for liposuction, but I must lose some weight first, so he referred me to a nutritionist. The surgeon had also advised me to adopt a healthy lifestyle and then go for liposuction.
> "However, I decided not to go to the nutritionist, but it came to my mind that if the surgeon wanted me to lose weight before going for surgery, then why would I have to go to him anyway? So I thought I should try your program first and save a lot of money.
> "Now, I am following your program that you gave me on my last visit, and it is working beautifully."

"Mr. Smith, I have been telling you all long to follow this program, but you refused. Now all of a sudden, you are following the same program. What made you change your mind?"

This is what he said,

> "When you used to tell me to lose weight, I thought 'Let me enjoy my meat and desserts, and one day I'll go to the surgeon and get fixed.' But now I can put everything into perspective and appreciate what you have been telling me all along. I see that the first surgeon wanted to charge me $5,000 which I could not afford, and the same surgeon told me that liposuction would not solve the root cause of my problem.
>
> "The second surgeon told me that he would charge less but I had to lose weight first. I can appreciate that I was wrong when I used to think that let me enjoy my food now, and later I would go for liposuction. I felt that I had run out of options. I also came to the realization (awareness) that a healthy lifestyle is the only and best option if I want permanent results."

He also told me that now he eats salad and fish, and feels great. He also told me that he feels so good that he does not miss any meat, dessert or bread. He also told me that also stopped drinking any soda. Before leaving, he said something in a joking manner, "Watch, Doctor, when I see you next I may be as slim as you."

I thought, 'Isn't it interesting how different people come to the same conclusion after going around in circles? I also understand that people are unique and have their own way of analyzing things. It is hard to comprehend what factor or situation triggers a change in a person.'

You have read several stories in this book, and you have noticed that in one patient, the change happened because he did not want to lose his leg to diabetes. Before that incident, he did not listen to my suggestion or advice. In another case, the transformation came overnight as the lady started to look at herself from a different perspective, although she had been looking at herself in the same mirror for years, and so on.

This story affirms my belief that I, as a physician, should never give up on any patient, no matter how resistant or stubborn he or she may be. I would never know what incident or thought might trigger the change.

Of course, it continues to affirm my strong belief that there is no replacement for a healthy lifestyle if one wants permanent results.

Story 14

Diabetic Cure – A Promise

Behold the power and magic of the self-kept promise!

This is the inspiring story of a man who was so devastated with the diagnosis of diabetes that he made a promise to himself that he will get rid of his condition once for all, and he did.

Mr. KS came to me in June 1998 for a dangerous infection in his scrotum. He was 49 years old, 6'7" and weighed 349 pound. His blood pressure was 160/100. He did not smoke or drink and denied any allergies. He stated that he had not seen a doctor in twenty years because he felt good and had no symptoms. He believed that he did not have any medical condition and denied any surgeries in the past, although he did admit that diabetes runs in the family. He was not married and had no children. He worked for a painter and was happy, go-lucky man.

When I asked about his dietary habits, I came to understand that he had no concept of nutrition. He never cooked at home. He said it was a hassle because he was the only one. "So, when I get hungry, I go to the shop around the corner and buy pizza and Coke or get burger and French fries," and according to him, "This has been my staple diet, and I have never had any issues with this it."

Regarding his condition of the scrotum, I learned after the examination that he was suffering from severe scrotal infection and therefore was hospitalized. Immediately on admission, routine blood work was done, and the diagnosis of diabetes was made in a matter of hours. His blood glucose on admission was 395. Scrotal infection can be very dangerous, especially if the diabetes is in the background.

In the hospital, he received aggressive treatment with IV antibiotics and insulin injections. After one week, his glucose was ranging from 200 to 250, and his infection was brought under control. He was discharged to follow up with my office. At the time of discharge: He was advised to continue with antibiotics by mouth and also to take insulin injections. He was educated as to how to adjust insulin doses based upon his blood sugar. He was also given education about his diabetic condition, and he also received two hours of education about diet and nutrition. He was cautioned that he must continue to follow it indefinitely for his condition because diabetes poses a lifelong problem.

He came to my office one week later for a checkup. At this time, his infection in the scrotum had almost gone. He was still hassling with his blood sugar, and it was not going below 200.

"Dr. Singhal, do you think I will have to take insulin injections all my life?" he asked.

I told him, "Yes, if you do not lose weight and do not change your life style."

"If I lose weight, can I get rid of my diabetes?"

I told him, "Most likely, yes, but I cannot guarantee."

At this juncture, he raised his right hand and told me, "I will lose weight and cure my diabetes. This is a promise. I was not aware of the fact that obesity can be so bad for me."

I followed him very closely thereafter. I checked on him every two to four weeks, and he was losing approximately eight to ten pounds per month. His blood glucose continued to drop gradually. After three months of treatment and observation, he was taken off the insulin and put on diabetic pills by mouth.

After two more months of observation and treatment, he had lost close to 49 pounds and his blood sugar had been come down gradually. I was able to control his condition with the diabetic pills only.

He continued to progress with the each visit; therefore, after another two months of observation, his blood glucose became normal, and I took him off his diabetic medications, although I still continued to follow him. I advised him repeatedly that as long as he maintained his weight, his diabetes could remain under control, but the moment he gained weight, his diabetes could return. He must continue to follow up with this office for a long time to come.

On his last visit, he said to me, "Dr. Singhal, how is this for a promise?"

I congratulated him and told him, "Yes, you kept your promise, and you did great."

I asked him the secret of his success. He said, "I am not very educated and I never went to college, but once I make a promise, I keep it. I was not aware that I had diabetes."

I saw him five years later for some other condition, and he still had no touch of diabetes.

There are two types of diabetes: Type I and Type II. Type I is an early onset type and is quite serious. It usually affects the very young, is fortunately not common, and is not related to obesity.

Mr. KS was suffering from Type II diabetes, which is extremely common and fortunately can be brought under control in many cases with exercise, weight management, balanced diet, and by eating plenty of vegetables. I have observed many times that vegetables play an important role in controlling diabetes. It may be the minerals, the enzymes, or even the bitter elements in them that may be responsible for this benefit.

Here I would like to stress the importance of vegetables and fruits for general health as well as for diabetes. Vegetables not only make the body alkaline but also are low in calories. They are very rich in minerals which have beneficial effects not only on general health but also in the control of diabetes. It is good to know that vegetables have some degree of anti-inflammatory properties.

This story demonstrates the power and the magic of the kept self-promise. I sincerely believe that human being can achieve almost anything as long as they are sincere with themselves.

Story 15

Can you save my teeth?

One Friday evening when I came home after taking my calls from the hospital, I experienced pain in one of my right lower teeth. I was an ER physician at that time. I did not think much about it, but in the middle of the night, I woke up with severe pain and had difficulty sleeping. I did not have any pain medication at home except Tylenol that did not help. On the rise of the sun on Saturday morning, I started to call one dentist after another but they were all closed till Monday. Then I prescribed painkillers for myself and went to the pharmacy to get them, and I got some temporary relief.

On Monday morning, I took a day off from the job and started calling one dentist after another to find who would take me first. Up to that time, I did not have my own dentist because I never had gone to one. Finally, after making several calls with different dentists, I was lucky to get appointment with one at 5:00 p.m.

I reached dentist's office at 4:00 p.m., hoping that somebody would not show up or there was a cancellation or somehow the dentist had finished his cases earlier. However, that did not happen. As a matter of fact, the dentist had an emergency, so my appointment was delayed for another hour. In that hour, I was praying that I do not have a cavity. The word cavity used to scare me because I know it is a painful condition to endure. I learned from my friends that the treatment of a cavity is a painful and long, drawn-out process. You have to go for drilling, then filling, and finally capping and so on.

At 6:00 p.m., I was called into the examining room. I sat in the chair for the first time in my life at the age of thirty-one. The dentist came and looked all of my teeth. He told me I had no cavity, and I took a big sigh of relief, but then he told me that I had a gum infection. He gave me antibiotic for that. He also warned me that I had a gum disease and that my gums were receding, so I must see a periodontist. Next, he asked me a question, which was quite embarrassing. "When did you last see a dentist?" I kept quiet because I never had gone to a dentist.

Let me admit that during my childhood, I was not sincere about brushing my teeth because I did not understand the importance of it. I used to brush my teeth not for the purpose of cleaning them but just to satisfy my parents.

In those days many people in India used a twig of a tree named 'neem' for the purpose of brushing. It used to take half an hour or so, and I hated that. I thought it is quite a waste of time.

On the contrary, many people loved brushing with the twig of a neem tree. It has two purposes. Firstly, it is very bitter, so it acts as a bactericidal or antiseptic, and secondly, since you have to chew it, it is very hard but it gives the teeth a good exercise. This is one of the reasons that most people, at least in the state of Punjab, have very strong teeth.

Now coming back to my tooth problems, I took the antibiotic and felt better. I realized that I had to find a periodontist which was not an easy a job as I had thought. I called couple of periodontists, and they recommended that I go for gum surgery for my receding gums, but I did not like that. I knew that one of my cousin's brothers also had a similar problem, and he went to periodontist who recommended the gum surgery which was a total failure.

Fortunately, in the hospital where I was employed as an ER physician, there was a residency program for dentists. I had become a friend with one of the dental residents over the years. I asked him if he knew a good periodontist. He told me, yes, but she was quite expensive. I said to him that was fine. He gave me the name of the periodontist, and I called her immediately from the hospital and made the appointment.

I went to the dentist's office as scheduled, and on the very first visit, she told me that I had a gum disease and that my gums were receding. If you do not do anything about that, you can lose all your teeth, so I became nervous. Next I asked her, **"Can you save my teeth?"**

She replied, yes. However I had to sign up for a five-visit program, and I agreed.

On my very first visit, she told me that the key to healthy and strong teeth is prevention and that means good dental hygiene. I was very impressed with her approach because I know from experience that doctors who believe in prevention know their fields best. To me, prevention is the king of all treatments. Next she performed a deep cleaning of my teeth. This was my first experience of deep teeth cleaning, at the age of thirty-one.

That was the day that I came to realize how important dental hygiene is and how I had been ignoring the care of my teeth. I made up my mind that taking care of my teeth would be my other priority.

On the second visit, she showed me the correct technique of brushing teeth. As a matter of fact, she brushed my teeth slowly for the sake of demonstration. She told me that my technique of brushing had been wrong.

On third visit, she stressed upon me the importance of dental flossing. She told me that people who floss their teeth regularly have very strong teeth. I asked her why flossing is so important?

At this juncture, she gave me a brush and toothpaste. She told me brush my teeth right there at the sink. I brushed my teeth to the best of my ability, and then I went back to the chair.

Next, she asked me, "Do you think your teeth are now clean?" I said, "I think so."

Then she told me that she would floss my teeth for two reasons: to teach me how to floss and why flossing is so important.

As she was flossing my teeth, some pieces of food debris came out that had been embedded between my teeth. She said that these food particles are cause of cavity or gum disease. She said it is impossible to get them out without flossing. She also advised me to floss my teeth preferably twice a day, but if I cannot do two times,

I must do at least once before going to bed, in addition to brushing my teeth at least twice a day. She stressed the fact that brushing and flossing are complementary to each other, and one does not replace the other. This convinced me of the importance of flossing, so I kept on with her recommendation.

On the fourth visit, she showed me the importance of an alkaline diet. She told me that an acidic diet is one of the important causes of cavities and gum disease. She told me that I must avoid all acidic foods—desserts, pickles, soda, sour foods, coffee, and alcohol. She also told me the importance of chewing vegetables and fruits because they are alkaline in nature.

On the fifth and the last visit, she again stressed the importance of prevention. She went over the program once again. She told me to check with her every six months, and I did maintain that.

Even as of today, I thanked that very periodontist who taught me all about the dental hygiene that saved my teeth.

This incident brought an awakening. I became more and more interested in dental hygiene. One of the important reasons was that I, as a physician, felt the duty to teach my patients the technique that had saved my teeth.

From there on, if and when I had the opportunity to meet a dentist, I asked them, "Tell me the secret to good, strong teeth." Fortunately, I have few good opportunities to learn from different dentists. In next few lines, I can give you the nutshell of conversations that I had with several dentists over time.

I asked one dentist how to prevent cavities. He replied, "Stop the plaque formation, and if there is no plaque, there will be no cavity. Cavities are formed only if there is plaque. On the plaque grow the bacteria, and bacteria cause the cavity."

I asked him, "How can one stop plaque formation?"

He replied, "Brush your teeth often. Ideally, you should brush after every meal. However, if you cannot brush twice a day, brush first thing after breakfast and second time before bedtime. You must also swish around your mouth each and every time you eat something, because lot of food debris gets caught not only in between the teeth, but also between the teeth and lips. The majority of the time, food debris can be removed by simple swishing around, but if not removed, it can lead to tooth decay and plate formation."

One dentist also told me that you can use your tongue to remove food debris from different parts of your mouth, or even you can use your finger for that purpose.

Then I asked the same dentist another question, "How long does it take for plaque to form?"

He replied, "As soon as you finish brushing your teeth, the process of plaque formation starts. However it takes fourteen to sixteen hours for plaque to be of significant importance. In other words, if you brush twice a day, you should be able to prevent cavities and gum disease."

I had one other opportunity to meet a professor from a different university who came to our hospital to give a lecture in the grand round. He shared that the more often you eat more, the chances you have of getting cavities. His explanation was that our mouth is kept alkaline by saliva which is very protective of cavities. However, whenever we eat, our mouth becomes acidic, and this creates an opportunity for bacteria to grow and cavities to form.

I also learned something very interesting from my brother Raj Paul, who is very fond of Internet search. I asked him how his teeth are. He said jokingly that his teeth are like iron. I asked him what his secret was.

He replied, "You need to know that your teeth have their roots in the gums; therefore, in order to have a healthy teeth, you must have a healthy gums. I rub his gums every day for five minutes in the morning and at night with my finger. This is called gum massage, and it is the secret of healthy gums."

Ever since, I have been doing gum massage as well.

Now let me summarize all the information that I have learned over the years.

1. Brush your teeth at least twice a day—after breakfast and the last thing before bedtime.

2. Floss at least once a day, but twice a day would be the best.

3. Massage your gum with your finger at least twice a day, two to three minutes each time.

4. Swish your mouth and teeth each and every time you eat. Make sure that you remove all the debris which is stuck between teeth and between teeth and the

lips. You can use your finger or tongue for this purpose.

5. Avoid acidic food, as much as you can and do not snack often.

6. Eat alkaline foods such as fruit and vegetables.

7. Chew your food well.

8. Squeeze your teeth often to strengthen their roots.

9. Most importantly, pay attention to your general health.

Remember healthy people have healthy teeth and vice versa.

Story 16

How a Man Cures His Own Blood Pressure

Mr. King is in my office for the fifth time in one year because he is suffering from high blood pressure. It has been quite a struggle for me to control his blood pressure, and there are many reasons for that. Firstly, he never keeps up with his appointments. Secondly, he comes in only after he has been out of his medication for a while. Thirdly, he continues to smoke two packs a day which has a negative effect on his blood pressure; and lastly, his life is very hectic, leaving him no time for relaxation and enjoyment.

I told Mr. King, "Look, I have not been able to control your blood pressure for a while; therefore, let me spend some time with you and try to understand your situation and your lifestyle so that I can be of help to you." He agreed to that. Thereafter, I had a long discussion with him and came to the following conclusions:

Mr. King is 45 years old, weighs 215 pounds and is 5'8". He is suffering from moderate to severe blood pressure. His blood pressure usually ranges from 170 /100 to 210/110. He smokes one pack a day and has been smoking for last twenty-seven years. As he said, "I started to smoke as a teenager under peer pressure but have not been able to quit ever since. I have tried nicotine gum, nicotine patch, and Chantix but without any benefit."

Regarding his lifestyle, he told me that his life is very hectic. He typically works six days a week, and if he is lucky, he can get one Saturday off per month. He further stated that he wakes up at

6:00 a.m., takes a quick shower, and leaves for work. On his way, he gets coffee and cigarettes from a quick store, as he has no time for breakfast. He also buys chips, cookies, and pretzels for the day. He has no time for lunch because he knows he would be on the road all day long. He usually gets home around 8:00 p.m., and at times even 9:00 or 10:00 p.m. when he children are already in bed. He further stated that when he goes back home, he drinks beer to unwind, takes a shower, eats a big dinner with his wife, and goes to bed. This is his typical daily schedule.

He further stated that his job requires traveling by car all day long. He works for a bank, and his job is to deliver money from one bank to another. He carries a lot of money, so he does not try to leave the car very much. He also told me that he does not drink much water because then he would be looking for bathroom all day long. He also said that since he travels a lot, he has to go through several tunnels in a day, and, as you know, the tunnels are polluted. That is the cause of his chronic sinus condition and nose blockage.

After listening to his story, I gave him a complete physical, including blood tests and EKG. After reviewing the blood test, I told him that his cholesterol was quite high. His total cholesterol was 230, HDL was 30 and LDL 170, his triglyceride level was 150. I also told him that he had no touch of diabetes and that his kidneys and liver were normal. His thyroid function was also normal. However, I told him that his EKG showed coronary ischemia.

"Mr. Young, you have high blood pressure and high cholesterol," I said. "Besides, you keep smoking, knowing that it can lead to heart attack and stroke, and you are too young for that."

He said, "Dr. Singhal, my family and my job are more important than my cholesterol and blood pressure. I have to feed my family."

After hearing his heartfelt comments, I became quiet for few minutes and then I told him, "Mr. King, I understand your situation better than before, but I can still help you if you will work with me." He said, "Yes, anything that is workable, I will do it." Thereafter, I made the following recommendations to him:

1. As soon as he gets up in the morning, at first he should drink at least half a liter of water. This will help him many ways. It will wash the toxins from the body and hydrate him; that in turn will help to lower his blood pressure and clear his lungs and nose.

2. He should carry a water bottle with him, not to drink large amounts at a time but to sip a little now and then. This will not make him need to go to the bathroom that much, yet it would help him to stay hydrated to a degree. I also suggested that whenever he makes his stop at any bank, he should use of the restroom so that he would not have to look for one when he is driving.

3. He should carry with him water-rich foods—apples, pears, oranges, cucumbers, broccoli cauliflower, etc., because the mineral content of these fruits and vegetables will lower his blood pressure. He also should not carry potato chips with him, due to a lot of salt in chips that can raise the blood pressure.

4. I advised him not to drink beer in the evening when he goes home after work, because that has a negative effect on his blood pressure. First, he should take a shower, have a cup of tea, and watch a comedy that will help him not only to unwind and relax but also to lower his blood pressure.

5. I told him to stop smoking, and this is must. This will lower his blood pressure a great deal.

I made an appointment for him in two weeks for a stop-smoking program based upon the schedule. In that session, I administered the one-hour stop smoking program, and fortunately, he has not smoked ever since. As you all know, smoking is one of the important contributing factors to high blood pressure.

Although I still see him very infrequently, and he still is not able to keep up with his appointments like before, but his blood pressure has come down significantly. He tells me that he feels a lot better, and now his nose is not blocked. He stated that now he does not have to look for the restroom while driving, and he feels quite at ease and relaxed. He told me that, under these circumstances, he is doing his best to implement all the suggestions that I gave him. He also confirmed that the stop-smoking program was one of the best things that he has ever done, and now he can sincerely appreciate how smoking was hurting him and how quitting smoking has been helping him.

I like to make a comment here. After treating this patient, I came to the understanding that although changing the habits and behavior can be difficult for some people, if a man off his schedule can make these small changes and adjustments to his life to lower his blood pressure, then anybody can do that.

There are several grades of hypertension: mild, moderate, and severe. It is important to know that most cases that fall in the mild to moderate categories can be managed successfully by simple lifestyle modifications such as stopping smoking, relaxing, eating an alkaline diet, practicing yoga, doing meditation, and so on.

You may also be aware of the fact that hypertension is an extremely prevalent condition in the middle and older age groups. It's etiology is multifaceted, i.e., multiple factors contribute to this condition—age, obesity, smoking, salt-rich foods, diet that is poor in calcium, magnesium, potassium, and other trace minerals, and of course lastly, the stresses and strains of life.

It is also important to know that one can have elevation of blood pressure as a result of the side effects of the over-the-counter medications which people commonly take such as decongestants, weight-reducing medications, nose drops, and so on.

Story 17

My Most Compliant Patient

Compliance with the medical treatment regimen is one of the biggest challenges that the medical community faces. It is frequently the cause of not getting the results that one has hoped for, and even at times can be the cause of treatment failure. However, the following story is about a patient who is compliant to the each and every word of mine (physician). In this story, you will appreciate the dialogue between him as a patient and me as the physician, and also how much he met his expectations.

Mr. William is in my office for his sixth visit, and it is time for his second annual physical. Mr. William is 52 years old, 5'9" and weighs 294 pounds. His blood pressure is 130/80, and pulse is 76. He does not smoke or drink. He did graduate from college. He is not married and has no children. He is a very caring person, and just for that reason he lives with his parents to help them, as needed.

As far as his medical problems are concerned, he has been suffering from high cholesterol, pain in the both knees, and obesity. In addition, he goes to the mental clinic regularly every month because he was diagnosed with some mental disorder. The diagnosis was based upon the fact that back twenty years ago, he used to hear voices.

I gave him a full physical, took blood, and took x-rays of both knees. The x-rays were normal. His blood test showed that his cholesterol was 294, which had not changed significantly in past two years, although he had been taking cholesterol medication. He had no evidence of diabetes or thyroid problem, and all other lab tests were normal.

There after I had a discussion with Mr. Williams about his physical, I told him, "Mr. William, your cholesterol medications are not helping you much. I can increase the doses of the medication, but I think if you can lose some weight, that will help you not only with the cholesterol and arthritis of the knees, but in many other ways."

Mr. William said, "Dr. Singhal, if you think I should lose weight, I will. I am the kind of person who believes that you must listen to every word of your doctor; otherwise, you are wasting his time. I also believe that if you are not going to follow your doctor's advice, why even go to him?"

He also commented that he was surprised that as of that day, no other doctor had told him to lose weight. "You are the first one to tell me. If you had told me this earlier, I would have done so. I am very thankful for your advice, and I will follow it to the letter."

I was amazed with his statement. I started to reflect why I had not I asked him before, since he had been my patient for two years, and I was not neglectful.

My reasoning for not asking him to lose weight at an earlier date was because I was aware that he was suffering from a mental disorder, and that he went to the mental clinic regularly every month. I thought if I told him to lose weight, it may add to his already stressed life.

Then what made me change my mind?

A month ago, I gave a two-day workshop: "How to be happy in life," and he was one of the attendees of the workshop. He participated in the workshop so actively that I was impressed with his thinking and reasoning. At the conference, I also came to the realization that not only he is a college graduate but also he has great potential. That day, I felt kind of guilty that I had been underestimating him, so I decided that when I see him next time, I will address the issue of weight loss.

Now, let's go back to the conversation with Mr. William.

Next he asked me, "Dr. Singhal, how much weight I should lose?"

I told him, "Look, you are approximately eighty to ninety pounds overweight, but even if you can lose thirty to forty pounds, it will help you a great deal."

"If you think I should lose thirty to forty pounds, I will," said Mr. William. "But how can I lose that weight?"

"If you start cutting down your food portions just comfortably little by little, you can lose up to one pound per week easily, and that could amount to fifty-two pounds in one year. That should not be difficult for you."

Mr. William said, "Dr. Singhal, you have to tell me how much I should cut down, and I will do exactly that."

After giving it a thought, I told him, "Maybe you should cut down your food portion by one third, and then we will reassess the situation in a month."

A month later, Mr. William came for his follow-up appointment, and he has lost three pounds.

I asked him, "How much did you cut down on your food portion?" He replied exactly one third, as you have told me. "Are you happy with my progress?" he asked.

I said, "Yes, you're doing great. Just keep up with the pace and do not go up and down with your weight."

Then Mr. Williams said, "Dr. Singhal, I want you to be happy with me, and if you think I should cut down more, I can. It is no problem for me."

I said, "Yes, if you can cut down on your food portion by half, it will be very good." He replied instantaneously, "That is no problem. I will do that exactly."

I saw Mr. Williams two months later, and he had lost an additional ten pounds from his previous visit, and I encouraged him to continue to do that. I also advised him to drink at least two liters of water per day. I also told him to walk couple of miles a day to help increase his metabolism and be good for his heart and mind. He said, "No problem." He was on disability and had nothing much to do in the daytime.

He came back again after two months. He had lost close to twenty pounds altogether. I asked him, "Mr. Williams, you're doing great! Let me check your cholesterol level again." At this time, his cholesterol level had fallen by only forty points, from 294 to 254, although I had expected a greater drop.

Then I said it was time to review his food diary. "Tell me exactly what you eat in a day."

"For breakfast, I usually take two eggs and toast with coffee, or oatmeal with coffee. For lunch, I usually like a tuna sandwich. For supper, nothing special as there is no regular cooking at home because my parents are not well. I usually take cold cuts or chicken and rice with dessert."

Next, I suggested that he should not eat meat more than once a day for many reasons. Meat is one of the most important causes of high cholesterol because it is rich in fat and calories. Of course, it is a different story for some people where cholesterol problems run in the family.

Meat is rich in salt. It is very poor in minerals like calcium, potassium, and magnesium. Although meat is rich in protein, he does not need that much protein at his age. Remember excess protein cannot be stored by the body, so if he eats protein in excess of his needs, it has to be eliminated from the body, and that can stress the kidneys.

I also told him that he should cut down on desserts, especially at night. He agreed to all my suggestions and that concluded the visit.

I saw him six weeks later, and this time he had not lost any additional weight.

"Mr. Williams, you have not lost any more weight. Did you change something?"

"Dr. Singhal, you know that I also go to the mental clinic. The psychiatrist at the mental clinic told me not to cut down on meat because I need protein. So I have not stopped eating meat. I also have to listen to them," he said.

Next I said, "I know my medical field, but you also need to understand that the psychiatrists are not the nutritionists. The diet which you have been following for so many years had not been helping you, and it was time to change, but again I leave it up to you."

"Yes, Dr. Singhal, I agree with you. I will cut down my meat intake to one meal a day. I'll see what happened. There is nothing to lose."

Two months later, I saw him again and at this time, he had lost ten additional pounds. He was very happy and excited. I checked his cholesterol which was almost normal.

"Tell me, why do you seem to be so happy and excited? Is there reason to it?"

Mr. Williams made a very remarkable statement: "Ever since I have cut down on the meat portions, my mental clarity has been improving day by day. This is one of the best things that have ever happened to me in years. Now I also do not hear as many voices as I used to, but most importantly, these voices do not control me, although they are still there."

At this juncture, I gave him a follow-up appointment at two months. Six weeks later, he came back and had lost another six pounds. He remarked that he had been feeling so good that he joined YMCA. He does not eat meat more than once a day. "Wherever I go, I boast how good I feel. Now my clothes do not fit me. I have to go to the attic to get my old clothes that I used to wear twenty years ago. Now I can bend down to tie my shoelaces that I have not done in a long time. I just feel great."

I saw him six weeks later, but he had gained three pounds. I asked him, "Is there any reason for your weight gain?"

"Dr. Singhal, I'm very sorry. I have just become lax on everything. My father is very sick, so I could not continue with my exercise regimen, but I will get on track soon."

I noticed that his statement was mixed with an apology.

I saw Mr. Williams after another six weeks. He has gained another five pounds. He explained, "I told you that my father is very sick, and that is taking a lot of time from me, but trust me I shall get back on track soon. I have done it before and I can do it now."

This story of this patient has made me realize that how a simple statement coming from a doctor, when there is a close doctor-patient relationship, can be so effective. From there on, I learned my lesson, and now I do not withhold any medical advice from any patient, whether or not I believe that patient could or would comply, although in some cases I may use softer language.

This new lesson has helped me to help more patients. At times I think I wish I had more of such compliant patients.

Story 18

Quit smoking in just one hour!

One Monday morning, I arrived in my office at 10:00 a.m., which is quite typical of me. (I don't start my office hours until 1:00 p.m. because there is so much office work and reading to do before I start seeing patients.)

Before I opened the door, I noticed a gentleman standing there. I introduced myself, and he said, "I am Johnny."

"How I can help you?" I asked.

"Can you really make me stop smoking in just one hour?" he asked.

"Yes, I do that all the time. How did you hear about me?"

He pointed out to the sign outside of my office. WALK IN A SMOKER AND WALK OUT A NON-SMOKER IN ONE HOUR.

"Are you really ready to quit smoking?" I asked.

He answered "yes" emphatically, so I let him enter my office, and we had a brief discussion.

(If the above patient had said to me, "I am not sure and/or I want to give it try," I would not have accepted him as a patient at least that day.)

"Johnny, tell me about you." I asked.

"I am fifty-two years old. I smoke two packs a day and have been smoking for thirty-five years. I started as a teenager under peer pressure. When I started, it was a cool thing to do, but nowadays it is a pain in the neck. I have to go out to smoke because the company where I work does not allow smoking in the building, and it is tough when it is cold outside. Also at times, my wife gets on my nerves about my smoking. I have tried nicotine gum, patches and even Chantix, but they do not work for me. I also went to the acupuncturist few months ago, and I was able to quit only for a month or so, and then I went back to smoking. I asked one of my friends who has gone to another hypnotherapist, and it worked for him. I have been passing this road every day, and I have been reading the sign outside that states you can stop smoking in one hour. I know that you are a doctor and hypnotherapist, so I thought I would ask you about the program. So I'm here."

"Why you want to quit smoking?"

"Because now I have developed emphysema, and I am at the stage where I cannot do any work without getting short of breath." He also told me that his son lives with him, and last week, his son's wife gave birth, and Johnny became a grandfather. "I am well aware of what secondhand smoking can do to others. I feel guilty about exposing my grandson to secondhand smoking. I cannot do that to him, so I'm ready and committed."

I accepted him as a patient. I gave him an appointment at 5:00 p.m. that same day. I assured him that by 6:00 p.m., he would be a non-smoker, and he agreed to come back for the session.

Just before leaving, Johnny asked me one more question. "What is your success rate?"

I told him, "I would like to say 100 percent, but in reality it depends upon the readiness and willingness of the person going through the program. You also need to understand that I'm giving you a one-year written guarantee which means I am confident that I can make you stop smoking in one hour."

Question: Is it possible to make people quit smoking in one hour? I have been asked this question over and over again. Yes, of course it is, provided the patient is ready and committed. I have been doing this for years.

Do I accept all patients who walk into my office for the program? Yes or no. It all depends on whether or not the patient is really ready to quit smoking. To determine whether patient is ready or not, I give every patient a brief interview, and if after the interview, I decide that the patient is ready and committed, and he or she is there for the right reason, I accept them. Otherwise, I tell them to come back when they really want to quit smoking.

I have learned from experience that when patients make statements such as 'I want to give it a try,' or 'I don't think I can quit, but my boss or my spouse are after me,' I know these patients are there not for the right reason, and therefore I discourage them from going through the program at that time. I tell them to come only when they really want to quit.

Although it has been my observation that the vast majority of the patients who come to me to stop smoking are ready and willing, however there are always some exceptions.

When you put Johnny to the above test you will agree with me, that he was ready and motivated. His reasoning to quit smoking was good and strong. Therefore accepting him as a patient was the correct decision.

Now, let us come back to our patient Johnny. He showed up at 5:00 p.m. as scheduled.

When people come for hypnosis for any reason, the very first thing that I do is to make them relax and educate them about the safety and effectiveness of hypnosis. I also try to give insights into their smoking habits as to how it had been hurting them and how they will benefit from not smoking.

Therefore, I explained to Johnny that medical hypnosis is a safe and effective modality without any side effects. I told him that I would not be touching him except his hand. I assured him that in hypnosis he would be in charge and in control of himself. There is no way in the world that I could control him.

(It is extremely important for hypnosis patients to understand that they will be in control during the session. There is a myth in the public mind that the hypnotherapist can control their clients.)

I also assured him that he could not get stuck in hypnosis. This is another common myth which I had to remove from Johnny's mind to make him relax.

Next, for the purpose of education and insight, I told Johnny, "You have been smoking for thirty-five years, and you smoke two packs a day. That means you smoke close to 730 packs per year (365x2). If you multiply that by thirty-five years, it will come to

25,550 packs. That is the number of the packs that you have smoked so far."

He was surprised and started to smile. "I never thought about it that way."

Next, I told him, "If we take the average cost of one pack of cigarettes as $8, it means you have spent close to $5,840 per year. And if you multiply by thirty-five years, it will come to $204,400. This is the money you spent on smoking so far. You could have bought a house with that money." After hearing my statement, he became more surprised and even more relaxed.

I also told him, that from now on he would be saving close to $5,840 each year, year after year, as long as he does not smoke. I asked him think about what he would do with that extra money. He started to laugh again. When people start to laugh, it is a good sign.

I further told him that money was not the main issue. "Look what you have done to yourself," I said. "You have difficulty breathing. You have to go outside to smoke during work breaks because smoking is no longer considered social. Most importantly, you now realize that, due to the dangers of secondhand smoke, you do not want to subject your family and your new grandson to your smoking."

He replied, "Dr. Singhal, I agree with you, and that is why I'm here."

Now I knew he is fully ready for the hypnosis. In the very first step, I hypnotized him. The hypnosis session lasts about forty-five minutes. I gave him a strong message that he was here to stop smoking once for all. Then I built his confidence during the state of deep hypnosis. I cannot give the exact words I used, but here is the essence of what I said.

Under hypnosis, I convinced him that:

*Smoking is one of the worst things that he can do to himself. It is not good for his health or wealth.

*I made him understand and believe that being a non-smoker is a beautiful new way of life that he is embracing today.

*I made him believe and realize that cigarettes are nothing more than cancer or emphysema sticks, and he cannot have them control his life.

*I also assured and convinced him that he has a very strong mind, and he can do anything if he puts his mind to it.

*I made him realize that today is the best day to take control of his life and behavior.

*Finally, I let him made a promise that he would remain a non-smoker for rest of his life.

Next, I took him out of hypnosis gradually. Immediately after the session, once again I reaffirmed the above statements that I had just told him in hypnosis, and that concluded the session.

I congratulated him and told him that his family should also congratulate him. Finally, he should congratulate himself for this bold step.

Then I taught him how to empower himself. I told him to make a list of all the proud moments of his life and his accomplishments and to think of those moments anytime the cigarette came his way. This would help him to stay strong and firm in his mission.

It was 6:00 p.m. I told him, "Now you are in non-smoker, and I have kept my promise to the time. Thank you for coming. I'm available for you for one year if you need any extra help. This is the part of the commitment of the program."

I did follow him for one month, and he had not resumed smoking, and every time I called him, he thanked me.

From my experience as a hypnotherapist and the physician, I know that STOP SMOKING is one of the easiest and most successful programs that any good hypnotherapist can administer.

Next, I'd like to cite a unique case from my practice. This is an example of an extremely motivated patient.

As soon as I took that patient out of hypnosis for the STOP SMOKING program, he said something beautiful. "Dr. Singhal, do not mention the word cigarette. It will make me throw up."

I was thrilled with his statement. I have on other occasions heard somewhat similar statements, but this was the best one.

The chief message of this story is that the mind is an extremely powerful element; it can do wonders. You can practically achieve anything if you put your mind to it. Hypnosis is just a tool that uses the power of the mind and subconscious mind to achieve one's goals.

I have seen that many patients even quit smoking "cold turkey." This is another sign of the power of the mind. In other words, if you believe you can do something, then you can.

I am often asked by people or my patients, "After I go through the program, how long will I remain in non-smoker?"

My answer is, "From my experience, the vast majority former smokers do not go back to smoking; however, there is a very small percentage of people who under stress or for some other reason do return to smoking. The good news is that they can be made to quit smoking again by re-administering the program.

Story 19

Dealing with Family Tragedy –
Two Deaths in a Matter of Minutes!

This was one of the usual yearly family vacations in the month of July at our favorite city, Rishi Kesh, a holy and spiritual city where there are also facilities for picnic and camping. We were all enjoying our weeks' vacation—having fun, playing games, enjoying rich food, joking, taking afternoon naps, and doing everything that goes with vacation. Nobody was aware what lay ahead of us.

All of a sudden, I noticed a swami passing by. He stopped at our camp and spoke with my father. The swami professed that something bad was going to happen to our family, and he recommended that it would be better for us to pack and go home. He made this statement around 6:00 p.m. In July, the days are quite long, and the sun does not set until 7:30 p.m. or later.

I forgot to mention that the on the previous night, my little nephew had gotten sick with diarrhea. He was less than a year old and was the youngest in our big family. No medicine was working for his condition, and he was going from bad to worse. All elders in the family were getting nervous; however, we the children had no concept of what was happening.

Now Swamiji's prediction made everybody nervous, including us the children. All of a sudden, sadness cast a shadow in the heart of everyone. Even on a bright summer day, it looked so dark.

I know from the past experiences that Swamiji's predictions usually come true. I shall give you one example. After graduating from college, I was struggling to get into medical school and was facing tough times. It was extremely hard to get into medical school in those days because there were only two medical schools in the whole large state of Punjab. As it happened, one of the swamis came to visit us at that time. He told me do not worry; I would be a doctor. I could not believe that the next day I got a letter of acceptance from the medical school that I had been admitted. I was just amazed how swami could know that.

I asked Swamiji, "How did you predict that?"

He replied, "It is not that hard. When you detach from the materialistic world and live in the spiritual world, you are on a higher plane, and you can see far into future and far back into the past."

He added that, for example, when you're standing on the ground, you can see only so far. However, if you go fifty feet above the ground, you can see much further into the horizon. Now just imagine if you go one hundred or two hundred feet above the ground, how much further you would be able to see.

Now we will go back to the story of our family. Influenced by the prediction of Swamiji and the sickness of my nephew, the family decided to end our vacation immediately. The decision was made around 8:00 p.m. that evening. The next morning, my father rented two taxis the size of large van, because ours was a big family—my parents, grandmother, seven brothers, three sisters, one uncle, nephew, and nieces, and so on. We were all young children except for my parents, two elder brothers, and of course the grandmother.

In one taxi, all the young children took seats. The only adult in our taxi was my brother, the eldest in our family, and he must have been near thirty. So, in our taxi, we were six brothers, two sisters, one uncle (my father's brother who was my age), four nephews and nieces. I was only thirteen years of age at that time.

In the second taxi were my parents, my grandmother, my second eldest brother, and his wife with their son who was sick; this was my nephew; the wife of one of my brothers who was in our taxi, one of my sisters, and three of our nieces and nephews.

We started our journey back home. It was approximately a two- to three-hour drive to our first target station before we were to make further plans. Both taxis started to race each other. Sometime our taxi would take the lead, and sometime it would be the other. Every time, when one taxi would pass the other, we made noises, waved our hands, gave flying kisses, and just had fun. Children easily forget what is going on with a situation and what lies ahead of us.

The time came when our taxi took the lead once and for all. We thought we had won the race. The competition had ended and the fun was over. Fun was in the game or competition and not in the winning. Finally, our taxi arrived at the first destination, the railway station, and from there we had to take the train. Unfortunately, the second taxi never made it.

We reached our first destination around 3:00 p.m. We were all nervous, worried, and concerned, thinking about what had happened to the family, and we could think only of the worst. We could not call anyone because there were no cell phones in those days. It was also not also possible to call even from a regular phone, not knowing where to call and what number to call. We spend the night in uncertainty, and, as you know, it is uncertainty that kills.

Somehow we passed that night at the railway station, but I don't know how. We wanted to cry but we could not because we did not know what to expect. My brother could not leave us because we were all children. You could see the anguish on his face. He paced the floor all night long and could not sleep. The children might have slept here and there, who knows.

Finally, the long and miserable night ended, and the sun came out. My brother fed us breakfast in a hurry, rented a taxi, and left in the search of the missing family. My uncle and I were left in charge of the all the children who were in our car at the nearby train station.

The discovery and the shock: One hour later, we saw two cars coming toward us. One was with my eldest brother who has just left. The second car was with my parents and everybody else who was supposed to be in the car, except two people, my grandmother and my nephew.

Miserable scenes at the station: My father came out of the car first. He had multiple wounds, all dressed, and there was blood here and there on his dressing. It made my heart sink and start to race. Next came my brother who was limping and had two splints, one on his right arm and the other on his left leg. He was already in tears because he has lost his son. Then came my sister-in-law who showed the anguish and pain of losing her son. Next came my sisters, and finally my nephew and nieces. Their clothes were partially burned because of the fire.

At this juncture, my father and my brother helped my mother to get out of the car, for she was in a bad shape. She had multiple wounds with multiple dressings all over her body. Everybody started to cry and kept crying for a while. We thought this was the end of the misery, but then my father spoke to my uncle (his brother) and told him that his mother has died. He was a referring to my grandmother. Next he told all of our brothers that our nephew has also died. Now we all started to cry louder and louder. It was a tragic scene at the train station. People gathered all around us in sympathy, as to what misery has taken over the family.

Although my father was in extreme emotional pain with tears in his eyes, he did his best to explain how the accident had happened. He told us that their car had fallen into a ditch and caught fire. The accident happened in front of a military post, and fortunately, a military person watched the accident as it happened. He called the ambulance, and they took all of us to a nearby hospital. Since the hospital was small, the situation at the hospital also became chaotic as they were not used to dealing with this kind of situation. However, the doctors, nurses, and paramedics did their level best, and they worked on us for hours and hours. During all this chaos and the painful situation, the doctor announced that two people had died in the accident."

Something positive did happen during this crisis. A military person came with my five-year-old niece who was not picked up by the ambulance; she had been thrown fifty feet from the taxi at the time of accident. The military person told us that he had found her crying alone in the ditch. God knows when she would have been noticed by some family member that she is missing.

My father continued, "As soon as the car caught on fire, somebody had the heart to rob me and took away my money. I knew what was happening, but I was totally numb and helpless, and I could not do anything. When we reached the hospital, I had no money. Therefore I had to sell my watch and ring in order to pay for the taxi to come here." After hearing this, we started to cry even louder.

One can always learn something from the behavior of the elders. When the elders saw us crying with pain, they forgot all their pain and turned their attention to comforting us. In order to assure us, they told us, "Thank God at least we are here to take care of you. You can imagine that the worst could have happened."

It took couple of hours to pacify all of us, and thereafter, my parents fed everybody something for the sake of diverting of our minds. Besides all the physical and emotional pain, the elders continued to try to put up a show that everything would be fine. This is the best they could do under the circumstances.

Now, the whole family took a train to go home, and we reached there at 11:00 p.m.

My aunt set up a first aid station at home: As soon as we reached home, the very first thing that my elder brother did was to phone one of my aunts to come and help us. He told her that there had been a tragedy in the family. She was, at that time, a nurse at the hospital approximately eighty miles away. She was not told that her mother had died, but she learned that as soon as she arrived at our home.

She came to us 5:00 a.m. the next day. My aunt has a heart of a great human being and an excellent nurse. She tried to forget the loss of her mother in order to focus on helping the surviving family. She realized that everybody was injured and needed her help, and so she became the medical person in charge at our home.

At sunrise the next morning, my father called in a doctor. He told him about the tragedy and advised him to visit our family at least twice a day or more often as needed to take care of all the injured ones. It took little more than three weeks before the physical wounds could heal.

Emotional wounds are a different story: As the physical wounds were healing, the emotional wounds were surfacing, and it was a major issue. Emotional wounds are much deeper and more painful than physical wounds and much harder to heal. Two deaths in the family in matter of seconds, the grandmother and the nephew: It was a big emotional loss to overcome!

My father requests the services of a spiritual master: At this time, my father phoned one of the Swamis and requested him to visit us as our family needed his help to go through the grieving process. Two days later, one Swami came. He was in his mid-sixties. He had a very pleasant demeanor and spoke in kind and assuring words. He had sweetness in his voice that could comfort anyone, and he stayed with us for seven days.

Healing of the emotional wounds: After his arrival to our home, the very first thing that Swamiji did was to ask my father to gather all the family members together one hour a day, every day, for a family prayer. After the prayer, he would give us a discourse and in his discourse, he spoke in a simple, easy to understand language so that even the children could understand. He also assured us that he was available to each and every one of us all day long. I remember going to him several times because I was very sensitive, and I used to cry more easily than the others.

In an attempt to keep everybody busy, he gave us one mantra. He told us that we had to recite this mantra one hundred and twenty-five thousand times. He also told us that it was a joint venture. He knew that no one could do it alone. He told my elder brother to keep an account of how many times each person recited the mantra and then total it. This kept the whole family busy for a long time. He was trying to keep our mind focused on something good rather than brooding over the accident. It was not a trick but a method many spiritual masters use to help ease the grieving process.

Q/A session after every discourse: After every discourse, some of the family members asked questions of Swamiji. I cannot recall all the questions that were asked; however, some questions and answers I cannot forget because they helped to heal the emotional wounds of the family. Here are at least some of them. You should appreciate the simplicity as well as depth of these questions and answers.

My father asked the first question. "Swami, why did we lose our dear ones?"

Swamiji replied, "Death is a natural phenomenon of life. Everything that takes birth has to die. Everything that is created has to end. Everything that has a beginning has an ending. Birth and death are the two sides of the same coin. The moment a person is born, death is written on the other side of the face. The only mystery is that we do not know when. God has kept that in his hand.

Then my father asked, "Swamiji, is there anything that does not die?"

Swamiji replied, "Anything that does not take birth does not die. God does not take birth and therefore does not die. Our soul does not take birth and therefore it does not die. You need to remember that we are the souls and therefore we do not die. It is only the body that dies, but unfortunately, many people get confused on this issue."

One of my brothers asked, "Swamiji, do the dead ones suffer?"

Swamiji replied, "No. Life has two components: the body and the soul. Soul is the master of this life. As the body dies, the soul departs and continues its journey in another body. To the soul, this body is just a vehicle, or you can call it a covering. As our body needs clothes to cover it, our soul needs this body to perform the action. Now as far as the body is concerned, it does not feel anything after death. This body goes through the process of recycling to be created again. Hence, the dead person does not suffer."

(As you might know, Hindus cremate their dead. After cremation, the body is converted into ashes that merge into the ground. People in India say, "You come from the ground and you go to the ground.")

My father asked Swamiji, "Explain the phenomena of rebirth."

Swamiji said, "Look, you are the son of your father in this life. You are also the father and grandfather of your children and grandchildren. Similarly, in the past life, you were the son of someone and father and grandfather of others, but you do not remember that. Similarly, in the next life, you will be the son of someone, and you would also be the father of your children, and also the grandfather of your grandchildren, and so on. This is how the lifecycle continues. This is what it is written in our scriptures (VEDA)."

Then one of my brothers asked, "Swamiji, how many times do we have to take birth and how many times we have to die?"

Swamiji replied, "As many times as you take birth, as many times you have to die. But a time will come when you will wash away all of your karmas, and then you will merge with God. Thereafter, neither will you have to take birth, nor will you die. That time, you will be liberated, and this called salvation."

My father asked again, "You have explained that the dead one does not suffer. Then why do survivors of one who departed suffer?"

"Attachment," said the Swami. "Attachment is the root cause of most if not all pain and suffering. The more attached you are to anything, the more likely you are to suffer, and conversely, the more detached you will stay in life, the less likely you will have pain and suffering.

"In families, people get attached to each other by reason of comfort, help, and emotional support that they get from each other from time to time, and that attachment becomes the cause of pain. Attachment to anything can be bad; it does not have to be just the family. You must have noticed that many people get attached to their money, others to their houses, cars, or clothing, etc. These people are very likely to go through similar pain when they have to let go of these things, just because of attachment. Pain and suffering are usually in proportion to the attachment."

Swamiji clarified this by an example. "During my school days, there was a boy in his class. He was from a very average family; however, one of his relatives was very rich. On one of his birthdays, his rich relative gave him a golden pen, and this pen became a curse in his life.

"Before he got this pen, he was a happy boy and very kind-natured, and also he was very good in his studies. He used to help other students out of goodwill. However, after getting the pen, he became a different person. He used to worry a lot about his pen, and he lost his pleasant demeanor. Although he used to be a giving person before, now if somebody would ask to see his pen, he would get angry. He lost a lot of his friends because of his new behavior, and also his grade started to fall. One day, he lost his pen, and that day became the day of misery for him. He became depressed. It was all on due to his attachment to the golden pen."

My father asked Swamiji, "Tell us something more that could help us to get over the loss more easily."

"Acceptance," said Swamiji. "One must learn to accept the fact. The sooner the better. Acceptance will lessen the pain and suffering a great deal. You have to understand that life is a mystery. It is not always possible to understand everything that happens in life. God's ways are unique, and at times, it is hard to understand them."

My father asked Swamiji, "I have so many children and grandchildren. Please say a few words of advice to them."

Swamiji addressed the children. "Children, this is not the age for you to worry or grieve. Leave this to your parents or grandparents. This is their problem not yours. This is the time for you to focus on your studies and enjoyment. This is the time for you to grow physically and mentally."

Swamiji reminded us that he had given us a mantra that we must recite to help us to become wiser and smarter in life.

This type of dialogue and conversation went on for one week. This was very assuring and comforting because it helped in the healing of our emotional wounds. Swamiji did his best to lessen our grief with his wisdom.

Goodbye to Swamiji: One week passed in no time, and now came the time for Swamiji to go back to his ashram. In the last minutes before departure, we all got together, touched the feet of Swamiji, and asked for his blessing. At this time, my father gave some offering, also known as Dakshna (a token of appreciation for his time) in the form of some money and a new set of clothes. Swamiji accepted the clothes with hesitancy. He said, "I do not need two sets of clothes I already have one, and that is good enough for me."

Thereafter, most of us went to the train station to see him off. It was a five-minute walk from our home, and on the way something interesting happened.

Example of the non-attachment: As we were walking, a beggar walked up to Swamiji and asked for some clothes. The beggar said that he had no clothes. Swamiji gave him the same clothes that my father had given to him as a gift. Swamiji said to my father, "He needs these clothes more than I do. Anyway, why do I need two sets of clothes?"

This touched my heart. I was impressed by his generosity and sense of detachment. Swamis practice what they teach. Maybe this was his way of teaching us about non-attachment.

The emotional moment: Swamiji had been telling us for seven days that we should not get attached to anything. However, I got attached to his voice which was very assuring and comforting. Before I could say goodbye to Swamiji, I started to cry. He told me in a laughing manner, "Pratap, I have been telling you all along not to get attached to anything if you want happiness in life. It is the time me to go back to my ashram, but more importantly it is the time for you to go back to your studies." He stressed that the primary duty of a student is his studies, and he must fulfill it.

The train arrived, Swamiji entered the train, and the train left. We came home with a heavy heart.

As a result of this tragedy, many things happened in our family:

> 1. The whole family kept busy for a long time because we were advised to recite the mantra 125,000 times, and this was not an easy task. I believe one of the purposes behind it was to keep us from brooding over the accident.

> 2. Before this tragedy, both of my parents and most of the elders used to pray regularly morning and evening.

However, after this tragedy, everybody in the family started to pray regularly. This had a great impact on life of everyone; even today, I do not leave home without saying my prayer.

3. My uncle, who was my father's brother and my age, became my best friend. He had lost his both parents, his mother had just died in this accident and he lost his father when he was a little boy. We were in the same class and the same school, and we studied the same subjects. We ate and slept at the same time. We were given a room in our home to share. We were best roommates for five years until we graduated from high school. We helped each other to study, and we both passed in the high first class. This was a big achievement at that time.

4. From there on, our family also started to pray together periodically at the advice of the Swami. Although we are a close-knit family to begin with, now we got closer to each other.

By the end of the year, the tragedy was fading away in mind of most family members except a few.

Swamiji is coming back: One day all a sudden, my father announced that Swamiji was coming back to meet us. This was a totally different situation, a joyous time, and we gave him a special welcome.

What a tragedy!

What a transformation!

You may remember the common saying, "What does not kill you makes you stronger."

Story 20

The Families in Distress – A $20 Cure

From time to time, I come across families in distress. Since I am the family physician in many cases, I know the entire families and have good insight into the functioning of these families; therefore, I have been able to intervene successfully.

There are different scenarios that cause distress in families. The cause of distress can result from lack of communication and/or misunderstanding. My solution in those cases has been to bring the families together and have an open discussion. That has worked in many situations. At other times, I see young couples fighting due to lack of insight into little things, and in those cases, I have the opportunity to intervene successfully by providing a little insight. Yet there are situations where both spouses are victims of a relentless busy life, and they do not have the time to see each other as both have their own busy schedules. In those situations, I often advise them to take a mini vacation, which has worked many times favorably to the advantage of the family. The following story is one such case.

I have known Mr. and Mrs. KM for many years. They love each other very much; yet at times, they become victims of the annoyances and demands of a busy life, and at times, they may even get on each other case at least temporarily. But usually they make it up with some repentance. This has been the trend of their twenty-one years of successful marriage.

Firstly, let me say something about the husband, Mr. K. He is fifty-four years old. He had been my patient for fifteen years. Mr. K is employed as a manager of a small supermarket, and he works six days a week. On the seventh day, he is busy at home doing odds and ends around the house—cutting grass, fixing broken things, paying bills, etc. He also has some health issues such as high blood pressure, headaches, weight loss, abdominal pain, etc. I think some of these health issues are stress-related.

Mrs. KM is a housewife and is very caring by nature, but her anxiety and nervousness are limiting factors, in that she is not able to help her husband as much as she would like to do. They have two sons and one daughter. The boys are in college and quite independent, and the girl is in high school and not mature enough to help her parents.

On a few occasions, when husband and wife visit together to my clinic, I have observed that there's a lot of tension between the two, although I know that they love and care for each other.

One time, I suggested that they take a mini vacation. The wife started to smile and told me that this was what she had been telling her husband for a long time. Her husband stated that he works six days a week to just pay bills. Although he is the manager, he does not make much money and therefore cannot afford a vacation.

"I understand that you cannot afford a vacation," I said to him, "but maybe you can spend one day a week with your wife, and on that day share your feelings with each other. This will make life less stressful for both of you, it may resolve some of the issues, and it would be also good for your health."

He said, "On the seventh day when I'm off, I have no rest. I have to do little things at home, and by the end of the day, I have no time or energy left for anything." His wife nodded her head in agreement as he made these statements.

My next suggestion was that maybe he could take one Sunday or weekend off in a month, if not a week. He agreed to that, but said he still didn't have money for a vacation.

I told him, "Look, you do not need much money for a vacation. Can you send $15 to $20 for a vacation?"

He replied, "Yes, that is not a problem."

Then I suggested, "Take a day off once a month and devote that day to your wife. In the morning when you get up, pack your meals and go for a picnic, or to the museum, or to a movie, or just bring the movie home to watch it together. This will help you to bond with each other more closely and make both of you relax. During that time, you may be able to sort out some minor issues in a relaxed manner. This may also reduce the anxiety issues of your wife and put a little ease on your stressed life." Mr. and Mrs. K started to smile in agreement and left.

I saw this couple again after several months, and I noticed a big change in them. His wife was less nervous and less anxious, and her husband was also beginning to gain some weight as he had been underweight. His complaints of headaches were much less, and his blood pressure was also getting back to normal. Before concluding the visit, I asked them, "How do you like your $20 vacation?"

The wife started to smile, and her husband's stated, "Yes, that is working well. We never thought of this before, and we both feel much better. Thank you for the insight.

As they were ready to leave I encouraged them to continue their $20 vacations. Both smiled and left my office.

I am sure you can appreciate from this story that sharing and bonding in a relaxed atmosphere can reduce lot of stress and tension between the partners, and money is not a prerequisite for a mini vacation like theirs.

I also believe that this case scenario is a prototype for several families and many can benefit from this.

Story 21

I want to live to be hundred years!

'Dr. Singhal, check me out good as I want to live to be hundred years," said AJ on one of his regular visits.

All of a sudden, my attention went to him. I smiled and nodded my head in encouragement.

Now, once again he repeated the same statement, "Yes, I want to live to be hundred years."

I said, "Yes, you can live to be a hundred years old, and it is not hard once you make up your mind."

Although this was one of his regular visits, it became very special after he made the above statement.

AJ is 85 years old and has been coming to me for last thirty-five years. He is 5'8" and weighs 132 pounds. He is married and has no children. He does have quite a few physical issues such as high blood pressure, coronary heart disease, cancer of the prostate, arthritis of the leg, and some cholesterol issues. Considering his age and all these conditions, I would say he is doing fairly well.

I examined AJ, took his weight, blood pressure, and pulse. I examined his heart, lungs, abdomen, and extremities. Today he looked better physically and mentally and was stronger in voice and tone than ever before because he was infused with the energy of his original statement.

What is unique about AJ is that he is quite balanced in his life and quite aware of himself and his potentials. He has a happy demeanor. Besides the physical conditions he is suffering from, I never saw him down mentally; he takes everything lightly. He has a very positive outlook on life. He and his wife are always together when they come to visit me, irrespective which one is sick. They are always making jokes of each other, even during the office visit. AJ is still very active in church and helps it in various activities whenever they ask of him. He told me that he does not worry about anything, and he believes in God. AJ reaffirmed his faith and said God has his own ways, although at times we do not understand.

AJ has been in the hospital a couple of times, and every time he had been able to pull himself out. He may not be in perfect physical shape, but as far as mental status is concerned, he is a good example.

I asked him, "What is your secret of being so positive and happy?"

"I take one day at a time," he said. "I do not think of the past; it is all gone. I do not worry about the future because nobody knows about it. I just live in the present and enjoy every moment of it. I do not question God. I have no right to challenge him because He knows best. I eat so little that my wife often remarks jokingly that I live on air. I eat only because I have to.

"I have never smoked in my life, I don't drink alcohol, and drugs are out of the question. I have no evil habits, nor do I overindulge in anything. I study something every day to keep my mind active, and even I go on the Internet every now and then.

"I like to exercise but I cannot because my arthritis does not let me; however, I walk as much as I can, even if I have to take several breaks in between walking. I may not be in perfect physical health, but my mind is doing okay."

I had few more patients who are long-living people, as you call them. They are between seventy-five is ninety-five. Although they have not made similar statements, what I have perceived is that they live with a somewhat similar philosophy. If I could categorize them and come up with a common theme, I would say: Most of them are small or average eaters; none are big eaters. That is in confirmation of the dictum that you dig your grave with a fork. Some of them smoke here and there, but most of them are non-smokers. Some exercise regularly; others are just quite active. Some are physically healthy, but some have few physical ailments.

Some believe in God, others do not, but all believe in themselves. Most if not all are pleasant to deal with; and none of them are complainers. The most important observation that I have made is that they all are mentally balanced, lead a balanced life, have a positive outlook toward life, and are quite content.

Story 22

The Moments Just Before Death

One evening as soon as I arrived home after attending my clinic, I received a phone call from India. I was told that my father had expired at eighty-eight years of age. I was greatly saddened by his unexpected death.

My younger brother and I left for India the next morning. At that time, I had been in my medical practice in the United States for close to twenty-five years. When both of us reached India, we asked our elder brothers who had been present at the time of our father's death two questions:

Firstly, did father have any pain, and secondly, did he have any wish?"

As a physician, I had been through many similar situations when patients die in the hospital after they had been sick for a while or have been suffering from a terminal disease. As soon as the family members arrive, they asked the same two questions: Did their dear one have any pain and did he or she have something to say?"

What I have come to understand from many years of life experiences is that the last moments are extremely important not only for the dying person but also for those people who survive afterward, whether or not they were present at the time of death.

The last moments just before death include the statement that one makes, whether one has pain or dies peacefully, and lastly, whether or not one maintains his or her balance in those moments.

The importance of the last moment also has fourfold meanings; namely, the truthfulness of the words uttered in those moments, the reflection of the person's life, the power and the potency of those words especially if uttered in anger or blessing, and lastly, if they believe in reincarnation that these moments will determine the type of next life one will be entitled to live.

In the remainder of this chapter, I shall elaborate on these four points.

Let me begin first about the truthfulness of the last words. You may or may not know that it is believed that the last words uttered by a dying person are true because the dying person has no reason to lie. This is true to the extent that the statement made by the dying person, if recorded properly through legal counsel, can be used as solid evidence in the court of law, even in criminal cases. Also the last statement of the dying person can be treated as his or her will, or may even override the previous wills, if and when recorded through legal counsel.

The last moments are the true reflection of the last few years of one's life. As you know, life is a continuum, and therefore a person's thinking, behavior, and demeanor do not change at the last moments because he/she is dying. Rather, people continue to behave in the similar manner as before. I can cite you few examples to prove this point:

You all know that when Jesus Christ was crucified, he said, "Oh, God forgive the innocent." This was the true reflection of his life. He believed and lived with that philosophy; therefore, he did not have to think about that statement.

You might be aware of the fact that Maharishi Dayananda was poisoned by his own cook because the cook had been bribed. When the Maharishi learned this fact, he called his cook and told him, "Jaganath (name of the cook), you have no idea what you have done. I have to leave a lot of work unfinished that I had planned for the benefit of the humanity. I advise you to run away from this country; otherwise people will kill you." Then Maharishi gave him all his life savings and told him, "This money is no good to me anymore, but someday it may help you."

These last words or behavior of Maharishi were also a true reflection of the life that he practiced and lived. He was one of the greatest Yogis, a social reformer, and one of the greatest humanitarians. He was in deep love with humanity. He had declared one time, "My life is not for me but for the entire humanity."

You also know that Mahatma Gandhi was shot and killed. His last words were, "Hare Ram (Oh God)." Again these words were the reflection of his life, and he did not have to think of those words.

Here is one another example from my childhood: My parents used to tell us that going to heaven was easy. They used to say, "If you can remember God at the time of death, you will go to heaven." Now I understand what they were trying to teach us. They meant that if you want to remember God at the last minute, you have to have faith and trust in God your entire life; otherwise it is not possible to remember Him just at the last moment.

Now for the third element: The words uttered at the last moment are considered to be very potent and powerful, especially if uttered in anger or as a blessing. Let me give you a case example from history in that reference.

Here are the last words of the dying parents, who were blind but died because of the emotional pain and shock when they learned that their only son has been killed by a king (hunter). Just before death, they cursed the king and said, "Oh King Dashratha, someday you will also die in grief of your son as we have had to die today." This story is taken from RAMAYAN, one of the greatest epics of India. Lord Rama was one of the greatest kings. His father's name was King Dashratha. The king was an extremely kind, caring, and compassionate person. However, he was also one of the greatest hunters and had the ability to shoot his prey from a great distance by just listening to the sound of it.

The story goes like this: Sharvan Kumar was the only son of the blind parents. He had devoted his entire life in serving his blind parents and he did not get married for this reason. One day, his parents expressed their desire for water as they were thirsty, and Sharavan Kumar said, "Here is the river. I shall fetch water for you." He went to the river, and as Sharvan Kumar put his pot into the river to get water, it made a noise. King Dashratha happened to be hunting at that time, and he presumed that an animal was on the bank of the river, drinking water. He shot Sharvan Kumar from quite a distance. When the king arrived, he could not believe what he had done. The dying Sharvan Kumar told the story of his blind parents to the king and then died.

Next, the king went to the parents of Sharvan Kumar and told the whole story and apologized for his greatest blunder. He offered them anything that he could do for them and promised that he would be responsible for taking care of them for their entire life. But the dying parents said they did not need anything, cursed him with the above statement, and died immediately on the spot.

This curse also was the cause of King Dashratha's death when his eldest son, Rama, had to go into exile for fourteen years.

Next, we come to the last element, i.e., the theory of reincarnation: According to this theory, the last words or the moments of dying person will determine what kind of their next life will be.

Our Scriptures state that life is a continuum. The beginning of our next life will not be much different from the life at the time of death, except we are at a little higher level. It can be compared to a student who graduates from one grade to a higher grade. Thus each subsequent life is supposed to evolve little more each time till it becomes close to perfection, and then we merge with God and rests in peace forever.

In conclusion, I admit that the information in this chapter is quite abstract and difficult, especially if you are not versed with the Scriptures. But I have tried my best to give you the importance and depth of the last moments of the dying person. I leave the rest up to you. You may or may not wish to explore further on this issue.

In this chapter, I have not discussed the obituary or the cremation or burial ceremony as it does not fall within the scope of this title; however, I do intend to discuss that in my next writing, which will be on the subject of death.

Story 23

Facing the death challenge –
I wish to die with dignity and in peace.

Let me begin this chapter with a case from my practice.

JH is an eighty-five-year-old patient who has been under my care for five years. He had been declared blind legally for a long time. He lives alone with the help of his neighbors who are very good to him. JH never married and had no children. He is intelligent and pleasant by nature. His main hobby is reading, although he is legally blind; therefore, he invested in a special machine that magnifies the print and helps him to read. He also spends a lot of money on books and audio books. Despite being blind, he always was neat and clean. His only other health problem is high blood pressure.

One time, JH ended up in a hospital for five days as a result of a mild heart attack from which he recovered quickly and went home. However, before the discharge, a pacemaker and defibrillator was implanted because of his slow heart rate and possibility of fibrillation.

Four years later, he was admitted to the hospital for the second time, and now he has developed kidney failure. A nephrologist was consulted who advised that JH needs renal dialysis. The next day, I informed JH of this fact.

Before I went any further on this issue, JH said, "Wait, let me think about it before I make the decision as to whether or not I want to go on dialysis. I'll let you know by tomorrow."

I said, "Fine. I'll be back tomorrow."

The next day, while making my normal rounds at the hospital, I went to visit him. I asked him, "Are you ready for dialysis?"

JH simply said, "No."

"Why are you refusing dialysis?" I asked.

"Because I want to die with dignity and in peace." Mr. JH continued to explain his decision. "I am fully aware what my choices are, and what lies ahead, whether or not I opt for dialysis. My roommate goes to dialysis every other day, and I see how much he is suffering. On the day that he goes to dialysis, he is very weak, and when he comes back he is even worse. He looks exhausted and is at the mercy of everyone. The following day, he recovers just a little, but the day after, he has to be ready again for the same cycle. He cannot breathe without oxygen. A tube goes into his nose which supplies oxygen to him, and he has another tube that goes into his penis. I cannot call this life or living, and I do not want to be dragged like him every other day. I would rather be dead."

Thereafter, Mr. JH was discharged to the nursing home at his request as he did not have enough help at his home. In the nursing home, every nurse knew that he wanted to die in peace and did not want any aggressive measures to be taken to prolong his life. He was put on DNR (Do Not Resuscitate) status. In the nursing home, he refused to eat or drink anything, including water. He refused even intravenous fluid. I visited him on daily basis, which I normally do not do, but he was a special case. In my mind, I believed that if he changed his mind, I should be there to provide timely medical help.

On each visit, I found him lying alone in his room on his left side. He was always quiet and never opened his eyes. He never asked any questions. However, on every visit, I would ask the following four questions:

1. Mr. JH, how are you? He would reply, "I am fine."

2. Do you need anything? He always responded by saying, no.

3. Would you like to drink or eat anything? Again he responded by saying, no.

4. Can I help you in any way? He would say, "No."

If I would ask him any further questions, either he would not reply or he would say, "I do not wish to answer any more questions." This went on until the last day of his life.

Once I was convinced that he was determined to die, I called the pacemaker company to deactivate his pacemaker/ defibrillator because I did not want his pacemaker /defibrillator to shock him at the time when heart would stop.

Finally, one morning at 6:00 a.m., I received a call from the nursing home that Mr. JH had expired. I attended his funeral and noticed that the word "Peace" was written on his face. At least, this was my observation.

The above case reminds me of two more similar cases that have come under my observation. Let me narrate them here.

The first case is of a physician who was on his deathbed, and he was one of my father's friends. My father was visiting him and I accompanied him. At that time, I had just entered medical school and did not understand much about medicine. His name was Dr. B and he was sixty years old. He had been suffering from high blood pressure for a long time; however, his condition had worsened recently due to very sad news. One of his sons, who was also a physician, had disappeared and was nowhere to be found. It was a great emotional shock for the father, and it might have aggravated his kidney failure condition. My father had a brief conversation with him. I do not recall all of the conversation, but even today I recall what Dr. B stated in a very composed manner, "Everybody has to die someday, and my time has come."

He showed no emotions while making that statement. I was amazed not only by his statement but also by his composer at that time. It was very difficult for me to understand the depth of this statement because I had never heard that statement before. My mouth stayed open and I kept looking at him. I still say that this statement came from his very depths.

As for the second case, it is one of my own distant relatives. He was ninety-eight years old, a truly wonderful man and a great personality. He had always been calm and collected, and this was his typical demeanor. When he turned ninety-eight, he decided to leave this world for good. He said to his wife, "It is about time to leave this world for a better life!"

All of a sudden to everyone's surprise, he refused to eat or drink anything. He lived for another thirty days and then died peacefully at home in the arms of his dear wife. What power and control he had of himself!

These are the cases that have come under my observation; however, I hear many similar stories. These cases amazed me as to how bravely these people deal with the challenge of death, and I honor them in my heart for a deeper understanding of life.

I believe that these people have very deep insight into life. They understand and accept the fact that death is inevitable and a natural phenomenon that everyone has to face one day or the other. They choose the quality of life over the quantity of just living.

The point that I wish to make is that throughout life, the perception of life and death keeps changing. A young, healthy person may be terrified of death. But an old, debilitated person who has been suffering from multiple health issues or who has a terminal condition or who is extremely depressed or, most importantly, people who choose the quality of life over the quantity may have a different perception of death. As a matter of fact, for some, death may be a welcome phenomenon.

Story 24

The best healing machine is yours for free!

It was one Friday evening that I was watching a wrestling match, and it was so competitive that I was glued to my chair till the match ended, which was quite unusual for me. The match lasted about twenty minutes or so, and it was one of the bloodiest matches that I ever had witnessed. Both of the players were injured badly and were bleeding. One person was so badly injured that he had passed out, the ambulance was called in, and he was put on the stretcher and sent to the nearby trauma center. All the spectators were in shock and concerned for his welfare. Some of the people were concerned whether or not he would make it. Even the announcers kept saying that the player had broken bones and difficulty breathing, and we all should pray for his recovery.

That night, I had difficulty sleeping, and I was wondering why these kinds of games are allowed in the first place. At last, I prayed for that injured wrestler.

Eight weeks later, I was watching the same show on the TV. I was surprised to see that the same wrestler was back on the stage, and this time he was able to defeat his opponent. I kept thinking over and over again how he could recover that fast.

Then I began to recall the stories that one of my classmates in medical school used to tell me. My classmate's brother was in the army, and he used to tell that at times soldiers gets so badly injured that it's a question of life and death. But when the injured soldiers are brought to the medical camp, with the all the best medical care, good food, relaxation and rest, most soldiers recover so quickly that they are ready to go back to the front for six to eight weeks. So strong is the spirit and healing power of the soldiers.

All the stories confirmed the teaching that I had had in med school: that our body is the best healing machine ever created by nature, and nothing else comes close to it.

Healing power is so deeply rooted into each cell, tissue, and organ of the body that the moment any injury or trauma happens, the healing process begins simultaneously and continues till the healing is complete and perfect.

Next, I would like to add one other extremely important fact: **This innate quality of healing power of this body can be expedited several fold by the determination and will of the person.**

Let me cite some examples to clarify my point.

You must have been amazed at the story of the patient who was suffering from terminal cancer and was approximately thirty-five days from death's door when he decided to pull himself back completely by just deciding that he was going to beat cancer, and he did within a period of several months without the help of anyone including his own doctor.

You must have been inspired by the story of a patient who had a severe infection of his genitalia and was on the verge of losing his parts because of severe diabetes, but by just making a commitment and promise to himself, he was able to get rid of his diabetes once for all.

You have also read the story of the patient who had high blood pressure and was not able to carry on his medical treatment and/or keep his appointments because of his busy schedule. But one day, I coaxed him to make small changes in his lifestyle, and then he was able to better control his blood pressure condition.

I wish to stress the fact that the healing power of the body is in complete autonomy **both at a local and general level, and this continues to confirm the dictum that the human body is the best healing machine ever created by nature.**

Next, let us try to understand the how the healing powers of the body works and how several external forces in nature contribute to the healing process.

For example, let's say a person's finger get injured; the hand has its own local healing system. The nerves, blood vessels, blood, and lymph of the hand come into play to repair the injury or the wound till it restores the finger to this original state.

Next, let us try to understand the role that the brain plays in the healing of the injured finger. The brain sends its own endorphins, increases the circulation of the hand, increases the nerve force, and stimulates the immune system of the whole body for the purpose of healing the injured hand, and thus plays a supplementary role.

The mind has its unique role in expediting the healing process too. The mind's role can be several times more potent than that of the body, based upon the will and determination of the injured or sick person, and of course that must have been clear to you from reading several stories in this book.

The faith and the spiritual element of the sick and injured also has an added beneficial effect on expediting the healing process. The stronger the faith or spirituality of the person, the faster s/he would be heal.

The blessing and the well wishes of relatives, friends, and especially parents helps a lot in expediting the healing process.

Now, let us also try to understand how several other external forces or sources contribute to the healing process.

Let me begin first with the five basic elements of nature, that is, ether, air, fire, water, and minerals. They all contribute to the healing of the human being, either alone and in combination. Of course, you must know that these five elements are responsible for the creation of the body.

Next in evolution are the plants or plant kingdom. Plants not only nourish the body and keep the person healthy, but the vast majority of conventional and Ayurvedic medicines and/ or homeopathic remedies come from the plant kingdom.

The mineral kingdom has its own contribution to the healing of the sick and injured. Many conventional medicines and homeopathic remedies come from the mineral kingdom.

The animal kingdom's contribution to the healing of the human is much understood because the remedies that come from animal kingdom are unique in the way that the emotional element in them is quite pronounced such as the feeling of love, hate, anger, jealousy, and so on. These emotional elements are not as pronounced in plant and mineral remedies. Homeopathy takes full advantage of this emotional element for healing the sick and the injured. Of course, these remedies are prepared from the animals of land, sea or air.

(You may want to know that the pharmacopoeia of homeopathic remedies is immense. Homeopathic remedies come from all sources such as plants, minerals, animals, and biological products.)

Our solar system also contributes to the healing process. The sun and moon have positive and negative forces to balance the energies in our bodies and therefore help to maintain our homeostasis or balance.

The power of community prayer in healing has been well documented as you will notice from the following example.

Approximately twenty years ago, a study was conducted in a hospital. In this hospital, patients were divided into two groups at random: Group A and Group B for a controlled study. A group of people gathered outside the hospital and prayed for Group A patients, but Group B patients were excluded. After two weeks of experimentation, it was concluded that the patients in Group A who had been prayed for did better or had a better outcome than did the patients in Group B, for which no prayers were offered. It was interesting to note that both groups did not know whether or not they were prayed for.

Now let me demonstrate to you a healing exercise which you will find practical and useful for daily use.

Exercise: How to use your energy for healing!

Bring your both hands in front of you with the palms facing each other, and close your eyes. Move one or both hands, a little at a time by only couple of inches going back and forth till you feel the push and pull force between the palms of your hand. Now hold on to this energy and let it build up. The more you focus on this energy, the more you will build it up. Next, apply the palms of both hands to the disease or the injured part for the purpose of healing, and do it several times. You will appreciate the healing effect. It is very simple to do. During this exercise, it is better to keep your eyes closed; but you may keep them open.

Let me caution you that if it does not work the first time, do not worry; just keep on trying. I can assure you that it will work, but it requires a little time and practice.

Now let me take the other side of the issue: You may be surprised to know that besides all the healing power being built in this body, some people continue to be sick forever and ever. I believe that certain people cannot take advantage of all the healing power that they have. There can be several reasons for that:

*No motivation or desire to get better

*Focus on the few benefits of being sick, rather than focusing on the benefits of a being healthy

*Ignorance: no concept of healing

*Extreme low immunity

*Trauma or injury too severe for the strength of the body to handle. However such cases are not that many.

Here are three cases, although they do not cover all the causes of slow healing or non-healing, but they do give you some insight into the situation.

Example #1. This is the case of Miss SV, a twenty-two-year-old female who had injured her right wrist at work a year and a half ago. She had been under the care of her company doctor for that duration and received physical therapy and other modalities, but she refuses to heal. I saw SV as a patient at the request of her parents after one and a half years of treatment had failed.

I asked Miss SV, "How are you? She said, "I injured my right wrist one and a half years ago at work, and it hurts a lot."

"Can I help you?"

"I do not think so," she replied. "My case is hopeless. I have received all kinds of treatment in the world, and there is nothing left. What special treatment do you have to offer?"

I asked her to let me try. I asked her to make her fist as tight as possible. She said, "I cannot because it hurts to a degree that you cannot imagine. You are just wasting your time."

I thought she was looking for compensation from work and therefore did not want to get better. However, later on, I came to know that this was not the case. The fact was that she did not like to do any kind of work and just wanted to sit at home and enjoy life with the television. As far as I know, it is past ten years and she was still on disability and had no desire, determination, or will to get better.

She was quite content with the fact that she is getting disability income and having fun watching television.

Example #2. This case is unique, but I see some prototype cases that can fall into this category. Miss GM is fifty-four year old and my patient for several years. She is five feet tall, but she weighs 307 pounds and is morbidly obese. She is suffering from multiple medical conditions, most of them related to her obesity. For example, she suffers from diabetes, high blood pressure, high cholesterol, low back pain, lethargy, and reoccurring current fungal infection, etc. Therefore she was on multiple medications. I have come to the realization that she loves to hear that she is sick, and also resents when she is told she is healthy.

On a few occasions, she came to me for something very minor such as a cold or an upset stomach. I had observed that whenever I tried to assure her that her condition was mild, and would go away by itself if she just gave it time, she resented my statement. "You do not know that I do not have a good immune system. You need to know that I'm a very sick person, and I do not get better so easily, therefore better give me antibiotics and pain medication and maybe even admit me to the hospital."

Conversely speaking, at one time she came to me because she was sick. I told her that she was sick and needed to be admitted to the hospital. After hearing the statement, she felt so much better that she started to tell me I was the best doctor she had ever known. "You are the one who understands how sick I am. If I would have gone to another doctor, they would have said there is nothing wrong with you."

At two different occasions, I ended up admitting her to the hospital because she was sick. On the day of discharge from the hospital, I told her, "Now it is time to go home." She asked me, "Are you sure that I am good enough to go home? Don't blame me if I come back. This is a good place, and people take good care of me. I'm in no hurry to go home. I have a good insurance. Let them pay and keep me little longer in the hospital." This is an example of the person who has no desire, intention or mood to get better.

Example #3. Here is a case of a sixteen-year-old boy who is a junior in high school. I have seen him five times in two months. Every time he comes with a different problem. All the work up on him, including blood tests, x-ray, and CAT scan of the abdomen have been done and negative.

The first time he came with a headache, he was hung up with the idea of brain tumor. Next time, he came with abdominal pain and was sure he had appendicitis. The third time he came with pain in the hand and was sure he had arthritis because his grandmother had it.

I have also observed that he did not like to take any medicine. For example, once I prescribed Tylenol to him, and he told me that he does not like Tylenol because it causes liver damage. At one occasion, I prescribed aspirin to him, and he told me that he is afraid to take aspirin because it can cause bleeding of the stomach. I have been in quite a dilemma as to how I can help him.

I believe the reason this boy is not getting better is that his focus has been on his sickness and the side effects of the medication, and not on getting better.

In conclusion, I can say that the body is one of the best healing machines ever created by nature, and most importantly, the healing powers of the body can be enhanced several hundredfold by the power of the mind and the spirit.

Although some ignorant or native people continue to be sick and not able to take full advantages of all the healing powers that exist, fortunately this makes up only a small fraction of the people. However, the vast majority of people continue to take full advantage of all the healing powers with which they are surrounded.

Story 24 ½

Half the Story

I strongly recommend that you should read this story after you have finished reading all the other stories in this book.

Why there are only '**24 1/2**' stories in this book?

The fact is that when I started writing this book my intention was to write 25 stories. It was also my wish that the last story should be a prizewinner. With that goal in mind I kept writing one story after another but none of them met my expectations. I kept thinking for days as to what I should do. Finally, a thought came to my mind that instead of writing one more story, I should let the reader write their own story. I know very well that all of you have a story inside you to share, and that could be important and even a prizewinner. Therefore I am requesting you to pick up the story and finish it.

Your story not only will give better insight on your life, but it may also help others.

The Outline of the Story: {Suggestions}

- It should mention who you are and how did you get at this stage?
- Also what obstacles did you face in life and how did you solve them?
- You can mention your accomplishment, and something you are proud off.
- The story should also have a message for other.
- The story should be a real and not a fiction.

Since it is an unfinished story I like to call it half a story.

Thank you very much.

Pratap C Singhal.

Questions and Answers

My Dear Readers,

Over the years, many of my patients have asked many useful and interesting questions. I am presenting them here in a Q/A format with the hope that you may benefit from them. I have also divided these questions into five sections:

A. General Questions

B. Question about Weight

C. Questions about Weight Loss

D. Questions about Food and Water Intake

E. Emotional and Other Interesting Questions

Section A: General Questions

Question 1. Why health is so important?

Health is your best treasure. Everything you do in life is for physical or mental health or well-being. In other words, if you could have everything in the world except your health, you would be at a great loss.

Question 2. How can you define health?

Health is not the mere absence of the disease; rather, it has a broader definition and connotation.

Health means whole. According to the *Oxford Dictionary*, health is defined as a physical and mental state free from illness or injury.

The best definition of health which is complete and covers all aspects of the human being is given by Ayurveda, the science of life. Here it is: "A healthy person is the one who is healthy at the physical mental and spiritual levels."

Physical level: In a healthy person, all physiological functions must be normal, the appetite must be good, and all discharges, including urine, stool, and perspiration, should be normal.

Mental level: One should have mental balance, which is indicative of mental strength and stability.

Spiritual level: One must be content and blissful.

Question 3. What do I have to do to stay healthy?

You must keep your batteries charged at the physical, mental and spiritual levels.

Physical level: Eat healthy, get adequate rest and sleep, and exercise.

Mental level: Keep your mental balance under all situations and circumstances.

Spiritual level: You must understand life as a whole, life is eternal, and anything which is material is an accessory to life. Therefore, in order to make advances at the spiritual level, you must continue your search for the bliss and joy of life, and not mere focus on the materialistic things that can provide only transient happiness.

It is also important to do meditation and prayer according to your belief system on a consistent basis.

It is equally important not to waste your energy unnecessarily at the physical, mental or spiritual levels. Overwork is a drain on your health. One must work hard but still keeping a balance between work and enjoyment.

Question 4. What is the single most important secret to health?

I believe practicing healthy habits is the key. We are the product of our habits. Healthy habits makes us healthy, and unhealthy habits can cause multiple diseases and miseries.

Question 5. How can you define healthy habits?

Being of normal weight, having balanced life, maintaining a positive outlook and attitude toward life. One need to know that, the healthy habits are the products of a disciplined life.

Question 6. Why is meditation so important?

Meditation provides mental and spiritual strength that is also reflected at the physical level. As an additional benefit, meditation also makes one calmer and more alert, and it can prolong life by as much as fourteen years.

Question 7. I have been very neglectful of my health. Is it too late to get back on the right track?

No, it is never too late. Remember your body is of a dynamic nature, that is, it is rejuvenating every minute of life. The day you start your healthy lifestyle, your body will remodel accordingly.

Question 8. Why is addiction so bad?

Addiction to anything means that the addictive element has taken over your life and controls you, and therefore you have become a victim and slave of it. The addictive element can be anything— smoking, alcohol or drugs, etc. To be controlled or taken over by anything is one of the biggest losses of oneself.

Section B: Questions about Weight

Question 9. What is my ideal weight?

Your ideal weight is calculated based on your height, although gender also plays some role. Therefore, there are different scales and guidelines for males and females, although the difference is very small. For males, a person who measures 5' should weigh 106 pound, and thereafter you can add 6 pounds per inch. For females, a person who measures 5' should weigh 100 pounds, and thereafter you can add 5 pounds per inch. You can also add another 10 to 15 percent based on your frame, if it is medium or large. You can add another 10 percent as a reserve. As a matter of fact, people who are approximately 10 percent over their ideal weight have more advantage than people who are of normal weight or are underweight.

Question 10. Why it is important to be of normal weight?

Because when you're of the right weight, every organ of your body (brain, heart, lungs, kidneys, liver) work at the optimum level. People who are either underweight or overweight are prone to have more diseases.

Question 11. How can being overweight affect me?

The more overweight you are, the more at risk you are of having high blood pressure, diabetes, coronary artery disease, cholesterol issues, GERD, arthritis, and even cancer. People who are obese also have decreased immunity, and therefore are also more prone to infections.

Question 12. How can I find out if I am of normal weight, underweight or overweight?

It is a two-step process:

The first step is to find your BMI. For your convenience, the BMI table is provided in the appendix that follows immediately after this section. Please consult the table before advancing to the next step.

In the second step, match your BMI with the following guidelines:

A. Underweight   BMI is less than 18.5.

B. Normal weight   BMI is 18.5 to 24.9.

C. Overweight   BMI is 25 to 29

D. Obese   BMI is 30 to 39

E. Morbidly Obese   BMI 40 to 49

F. Super obese   BMI 50 to 59

Question 13. Am I eating too much or too little or just right?

If you are gaining weight and you do not wish to, most likely you are eating too much. But if you are losing weight and you do not wish to, most likely you are eating too little. However, if you are not losing or gaining, and you are happy with your weight, or you are of ideal weight, then you are eating the right amount. This is a general guideline because at times, other factors fall into this equation such as a hormonal condition or an imbalance, fluid retention, etc.

Question 14. Can you explain the two types of body fat?

Yes, the body has two types of fat—central fat and peripheral fat. Both fats are bad, but central fat is much more harmful than the peripheral fat. Central fat is the one that collects around your belly. It can be measured by the abdominal girth or waist measurement that is taken at the umbilicus and not below or above it. Peripheral fat is the one that collects around the peripheral parts of the body such as buttocks, shoulders, extremities, etc. It is measured by BMI.

Question 15. How and why do people gain or lose weight?

It is a function of caloric balance or imbalance. In other words, if you take in more calories than you burn, then you will gain weight; conversely, if you take less calories than you burn then you will lose weight and so on.

Question 16. Everybody is fat in my family. Will I also be fat?

No, obesity is not based upon genetics or heredity. It is based on habits and lifestyle. If everybody is overweight in your family, it means they do not have healthy habits. You will be product of your habits, not those of your family.

Section C: Question about Weight Loss

Question 17. At what rate I should lose weight?

It will depend on how fast you wish to lose weight. If you work at a normal pace and lose about five hundred calories per day, which is really small, you can still lose one pound per week, and that can add up to fifty-two pounds of weight loss per year. However, if you go on a fasting diet, you can lose up to one pound per day.

Read the story of the two medical residents in this book, and also the story of a lady who traveled seventy miles per day.

Question 18. What are the best foods for weight loss?

Foods that are rich in water content such as vegetables and fruits are the best for this purpose. Vegetables are still number one, and fruits are number two. Vegetables are not only rich in the nine essential ingredients of food but also very low in calories. Vegetables are also classified as free foods. That means you can eat as much as you like without getting fat. (And I like that.)

Question 19. Are there any effective magic pills or diets for weight loss?

No. Magic pills and diets do not work for a long period of time. So if you do want permanent results, you have to get rid of your unhealthy habits and adopt a healthy lifestyle.

Question 20. Are water pills good for weight loss?

No. Water pills can help you lose water, not weight. Water pills can be bad for you because you may get dehydrated. The water content of the body is between 65 to 70 percent during good health. By taking water pills, you may be able to lose few pound of water and not fat. Is it worth the risk?

Question 21. Can eating slowly and chewing your food well help me to lose weight?

Yes. When you eat slowly and chew your food well, you will be satisfied more easily and will eat less. In this reference, read the chapter *The Best Peanut Ever*.

Question 22. Can an all fruit diet help me to lose weight?

Yes, this is quite an effective technique. I have used it on several of my patients.

Question 23. What is the best time for grocery shopping?

Studies have shown that the best time for the grocery shopping is after a meal, because when you are not hungry, you will be less tempted for the wrongful foods, and therefore you are likely to make better choices and come home with healthy groceries.

Question 24. What is the role of exercise in weight loss?

The amount of calories you burn in exercise is so small that it cannot be used as a tool for weight loss. However, exercise is strongly recommended for everyone, whether underweight, normal weight or overweight. Exercise is one of the best tools to stay healthy.

Question 25. I am always hungry. I don't know what to do.

My friend, you are in luck. A good appetite is a sign of good health. If you do not wish to gain weight, eat plenty of vegetables whenever you want and as much as you want, and you will not gain weight.

Question 26. Whenever I go to a party or buffet, I end up overeating and feel bad. What should I do?

Here are some of the suggestions that can fix your problems:

> Yell at yourself very loudly for doing so. (Just kidding.)

> For the next twenty-four hours, either don't eat anything or just eat vegetables.

> The following day, eat fruits all day. This should fix the problem at least for that time. Also let this incident be a lesson for future so that you do not repeat it.

Question 27. Is overeating okay at parties or buffets?

Yes, but then you must be prepared to make up for it the following day, as it has been discussed in the previous question.

Section D: Questions about Food and Water

Question 28. What is the importance of food in maintaining good health?

Your physical body is the product of the food you eat, and hence healthy food means a healthy body and vice versa. Conversely, one needs to know that what food is to the body, thoughts are to the mind. Therefore, for a healthy mind, it is important to have good and positive thoughts.

Question 29. It is well known that different foods have different caloric values. Can you comment on that?

Yes, caloric value varies from food to food. Let me give you some rundown of the foods. Let me start with the foods that have lowest caloric value and then go to foods that have highest caloric value.

A. Vegetables are the foods with the lowest caloric values and that have all nine essential ingredients of a food, which is why they are so great.

B. Fruits are as good as vegetables but have slightly more caloric value. Fruits also have the nine essential ingredients of a food yet are still low in calories.

C. Beans and grains have reasonably good amounts of calories and are rich in proteins, minerals, and vitamins, and are also healthy foods. However, you must make sure that you're taking the whole grain, for example, whole wheat, brown rice, etc., and eating them in moderation.

D. Milk and diary are next in line.

E. Meats are very high in caloric value and also rich in protein, but very rich in fat, cholesterol, and salt.

F. Desserts, carbonated beverages, and alcohol are foods of highest caloric value and many empty calories, and therefore are classified as junk food.

Question 30. Are carbohydrates bad for you?

Of course not. Carbohydrates are not only good for you but necessary for the functioning of the brain. The average person needs at least 130g of carbohydrates per day, but you must understand the type of carbohydrates that you are ingesting. Carbohydrates are of two kinds—simple and complex. Your goal should be to use as many complex carbohydrates as possible and to avoid simple carbohydrates.

A. Examples of complex carbohydrates are whole grain bread, brown rice, roasted beans, whole wheat pasta, etc.

B. Avoid all refined carbohydrates such as white sugar, white bread, white rice, pasta, and pizza.

It has been known to the ancient health providers that one should try to avoid carbohydrates with meat. So when you eat fish, chicken, cold cuts, etc., eat them without bread or potatoes.

Question 31. What do you think of meat as a food?

Meat is like any other food. It has plus and negative qualities. Let us analyze. The positive quality of meat is that it is rich in protein.

Some of the negative qualities:

A. It is very rich in fat and salt.

B. It is very poor in minerals—potassium, calcium, magnesium, and trace minerals.

C. It is very poor in enzyme content.

D. It is a concentrated food and therefore very rich in fat and calories. The fat content of the meat is responsible for raising the cholesterol level.

E. It is very acidic in nature.

There are some emotional issues as well about eating meat as it involves killing of the animals. Interestingly, one of my patients wondered why we put food (meat) into our body that has a lower level of DNA. In addition, I have also discussed in my previous book that man's body resembles that of a herbivore and not that of a carnivore. Therefore, I believe one should not eat meat or at least eat it very sparingly. This is also the recommendation of macrobiotics, the science of long living.

Question 32. How much water should I drink?

I would say to drink a lot without drowning yourself in it. (Just kidding.) Most people are dehydrated. It is extremely rare that one drinks more water than one needs, and I have seen only one or two cases in all fifty years of clinical practice. However, it is good to know that drinking water in excess of your need can have a negative effect on your kidney. Let me stress once again that most people are dehydrated. Now coming back to the question about how much water you need to drink on daily basis. It is extremely hard to lump all human beings into one category. The water needs of every person varies, based upon several factors, such as:

> A. Body size and body weight: The bigger a person is and the more one weighs, the more the water needs of that person. People who are underweight or children do not need that much water.

> B. Metabolism: The higher the metabolism, the greater the need for water.

> C. Climate and season: The warmer the climate you live in, the more the water you would need. Of course in a colder climate, you would need less water. It is equally true that in summer, you need more water than in winter.

> D. Activity: The more active you are, the more water you need.

> E. Perspiration: The more you perspire, the more water you need.

F. Food type: If you eat more solid and concentrated food—meat, dessert, fried food, dried food, salty food, sweet food—you need a lot more water. On the contrary, if you eat foods that are rich in water content such as vegetables and fruit you will need less water.

G. Medical condition: If you have a medical condition in which you retain water, you have to be careful how much you drink. In those cases, you must follow the advice of your doctor.

H. Thirst: This can be a very good guide as to how much water you need.

As you can see, it is hard to put all people into one category. Let me quote one authority with whom I agree. Nessler states: "In general, you should try to drink between half to an ounce of water per each pound of bodyweight, per day." Another guide that I follow it is to look at the quality and quantity of the urine. If you are urinating too often and it is colorless, it means your drinking too much. However if you are not urinating enough and your urine is too concentrated it means you are not drinking enough.

Question 33. What are the nine essential attributes or qualities of the food?

Foods can be analyzed based upon the following nine qualities:

A. Carbohydrates
B. Proteins
C. Fat
D. Water content
E. Mineral content
F. Fiber content
G. Caloric value
H. Enzyme and/or vitamin content
I. Acidic or alkaline nature of the food

Always keep in mind that fruits and vegetables are the only foods that have all the nine qualities.

Question 34. What are the various food groups?

These are as follows:

> Fruits
> Vegetables
> Grains
> Beans and Legumes
> Seed and Nuts
> Milk and Dairy
> Eggs and Poultry
> Meat

Question 35. Can you discuss the classification of foods based on the medical science of Ayurveda?

The science of Ayurveda has classified all foods into six categories based upon how the food tastes. It does not take into consideration the protein, carbohydrate, fat, mineral, or water content of the food because these are not important criteria based upon the science. The six classifications of food are:

> Salty
> Sweet
> Sour
> Pungent
> Bitter
> Astringent

This is a practical as well as a useful classification. The reason is that in Ayurveda medical science, diet is an important ingredient of almost every prescription.

Question 36. You have mentioned in your previous book that fasting can save your life. Can you comment on that?

Dr. Shelton, the founder of fasting, coined this statement. It is as true today as it was when it was initially coined. Fasting not only purifies and cleanses the body but also strengthens the person at his or her physical, mental, and spiritual levels.

Question.37. Can fasting be used for weight loss?

Yes, it is quite an effective modality for rapid weight loss. You can read the chapter *The Lady Who Traveled 70 Miles Per Day.*

Question 38. Are there several modified techniques of fasting?

Yes, there are several modified techniques of fasting. For example, water fast, milk fast, fruit fast etc.

Question 39. Is fasting safe?

Yes, fasting is 100 percent safe, unless it is prolonged and done too often. In those cases, it can be a cause of malnourishment.

Question 40. What is the difference between fasting and starvation?

Fasting and starvation are two different entities, and there is no comparison. Fasting is not starvation, and starvation is not fasting. In fasting, you're in charge and in control of your behavior and the program. Starvation is kind of forced upon you or you are the victim of the situation.

Question 41. For how long should the fasting be done?

It depends on your goal and your needs. It can be as little as eight to twelve hours, or it can be as long as a month. There are no hard and fast rules. In general, many people fast one day a week to keep their body clean and their mind strong. It is a healthy practice and I endorse it.

Section #E. Emotional and Other Interesting Questions

Question 42. Some of my patients have stated that they just look at food and get fat. Can this be true?

This is a pure myth. Most people think they need to eat three meals a day as they did when they were teenagers. With advancing age and decreased activity, you need less and less food. You cannot gain weight without eating food in excess of your body's needs. I often also say jokingly, if a person can get fat by looking at the foods, then how are there food shortages? People would stand in a line and look at the food and go home satisfied.

Question 43. Many of my patients say, "I'm not fat. It is all air."

Air does not weigh that much. If you are filled with the air, you may be ballooned out but not overweight.

Question 44. Some people say I am so busy taking care of my family, I do not have time to take care of myself.

Again, it is one of the myths of which a person is a victim. Eating healthy and eating less does not require any extra effort. If you are feeding your family and children healthy food, you can eat the same, and no extra work should be involved.

Question 45. There are times when I cannot decide whether or not I should eat.

When you are not sure whether or not you are hungry, it means you are just tossing between hungry and not hungry. You can be assured that by not eating, you will be doing a favor to yourself.

Question 46. Is being overweight or fat a crime or illegal?

I have just checked the laws of the country at the time of writing this book. To my knowledge being fat is neither a crime nor is it illegal. You cannot be punished or prosecuted for that. However, you may be punishing yourself, but no one else can or will.

Appendix

Body Mass Index Table

	Normal						Overweight					Obese										Extreme Obesity														
BMI	19	20	21	22	23	24	25	26	27	28	29	30	31	32	33	34	35	36	37	38	39	40	41	42	43	44	45	46	47	48	49	50	51	52	53	54
Height (inches)																	Body Weight (pounds)																			
58	91	96	100	105	110	115	119	124	129	134	138	143	146	153	158	162	167	172	177	181	186	191	196	201	205	210	215	220	224	229	234	239	244	248	253	258
59	94	99	104	109	114	119	124	128	133	138	143	148	153	158	163	168	173	178	183	188	193	198	203	208	212	217	222	227	232	237	242	247	252	257	262	267
60	97	102	107	112	118	123	128	133	138	143	148	153	158	163	168	174	178	184	189	194	199	204	209	215	220	225	230	235	240	245	250	255	261	266	271	276
61	100	106	111	116	122	127	132	137	143	148	153	158	164	169	174	180	185	190	195	201	206	211	217	222	227	232	238	243	248	254	259	264	269	275	280	285
62	104	109	115	120	126	131	136	142	147	153	158	164	169	175	180	186	191	196	202	207	213	218	224	229	235	240	246	251	256	262	267	273	278	284	289	295
63	107	113	118	124	130	135	141	146	152	158	163	169	175	180	186	191	197	203	208	214	220	225	231	237	242	248	254	259	265	270	278	282	287	293	299	304
64	110	116	122	128	134	140	145	151	157	163	169	174	180	186	192	197	204	209	215	221	227	232	238	244	250	256	262	267	273	279	285	291	296	302	308	314
65	114	120	126	132	138	144	150	156	162	168	174	180	186	192	198	204	210	216	222	228	234	240	246	252	258	264	270	276	282	288	294	300	306	312	318	324
66	118	124	130	136	142	148	155	161	167	173	179	186	192	198	204	210	216	223	229	235	241	247	253	260	266	272	278	284	291	297	303	309	316	322	328	334
67	121	127	134	140	146	153	159	166	172	178	185	191	198	204	211	217	223	230	236	242	249	255	261	268	274	280	287	293	299	306	312	319	325	331	338	344
68	125	131	138	144	151	158	164	171	177	184	190	197	203	210	216	223	230	236	243	249	256	262	269	276	282	289	295	302	308	315	322	328	335	341	348	354
69	128	135	142	149	155	162	169	176	182	189	196	203	209	216	223	230	236	243	250	257	263	270	277	284	291	297	304	311	318	324	331	338	345	351	358	365
70	132	139	146	153	160	167	174	181	188	195	202	209	216	222	229	236	243	250	257	264	271	278	285	292	299	306	313	320	327	334	341	348	355	362	369	376
71	136	143	150	157	165	172	179	186	193	200	208	215	222	229	236	243	250	257	265	272	279	286	293	301	308	315	322	329	338	343	351	358	365	372	379	386
72	140	147	154	162	169	177	184	191	199	206	213	221	228	235	242	250	258	265	272	279	287	294	302	309	316	324	331	338	346	353	361	368	375	383	390	397
73	144	151	159	166	174	182	189	197	204	212	219	227	235	242	250	257	265	272	280	288	295	302	310	318	325	333	340	348	355	363	371	378	386	393	401	408
74	148	155	163	171	179	186	194	202	210	218	225	233	241	249	256	264	272	280	287	295	303	311	319	326	334	342	350	358	365	373	381	389	396	404	412	420
75	152	160	168	176	184	192	200	208	216	224	232	240	248	256	264	272	279	287	295	303	311	319	327	335	343	351	359	367	375	383	391	399	407	415	423	431
76	156	164	172	180	189	197	205	213	221	230	238	246	254	263	271	279	287	295	304	312	320	328	336	344	353	361	369	377	385	394	402	410	418	426	435	443

Source: Adapted from Clinical Guidelines on the Identification, Evaluation, and Treatment of Overweight and Obesity in Adults: The Evidence Report.

To find your BMI

Plot your height in inches against your weight in pounds.

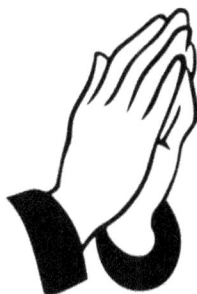

Until Next Time [Namastee]

I hope that reading this book was an inspiring and a rewarding experience for you, and that you had fun and excitement at the same time. You also must have realized that you have enriched yourself with a lot of practical and useful information, and you might have found the solution to your disease.

Another important point that I want to make is, more the information you apply, the more benefits you will get and the more you will be inspired, and therefore, the more likely you will continue to use this information. This, in turn, will create a positive upward spiral that will help you achieve your goals/dreams.

At this juncture I would like to ask you has this book inspired you enough to write your own life story, if so please do so, it will help not only you but it can also help others. This is what I had mentioned in the introduction and that would be the 25th story.

I would like to take the opportunity to make a suggestion; that is, if you sincerely believe that this book has benefited you, please do not put this book back on your bookshelf. Share, help, and inspire others whom you love or respect. It could be anyone or everyone based upon your friendships or social circles. It could be your own spouse, friends, colleague, doctor or priest, teacher or student, or anyone else. You may even think of giving this book as a gift to them on their birthday, Valentine's Day, Christmas, New Year's Day, and so on. Perhaps you might like to donate this book to your local library for the benefit of others. If you are a spiritual person, you know that giving in one way is receiving in another way.

Lastly, I wish to thank you very much for giving me the opportunity to serve you. I hope to meet you again in one of my next books or other programs.

Pratap C. Singhal MD

PS: You are also welcome to post your comment on Amazon or Barnes & Noble's.

Books by the Author

Health, Happiness and You – Everything You Need to Know
Available in paperback and e-book

Live Healthier and Live Happier, with the help of 101+
suggestions, formulas, poems, mantras and lessons learned from
short stories. Only paperback

One Solution to Many Diseases, presented in twenty-four stories
Paperback and e-book

Upcoming Books

Death – Who should fear it?

The Pathways to Happiness

Make me younger by the day.

Cancer-How to protect yourself

Meditation

Hypertension

Book Availability

Amazon.com

BarnesandNoble.com

Pratap C. Singhal MD, 431 Washington Ave Belleville, NJ 07109-2618

Or order from any bookstore near you.

www.ingramcontent.com/pod-product-compliance
Lightning Source LLC
Chambersburg PA
CBHW072129020426
42334CB00018B/1724